The
High
Blood
Pressure

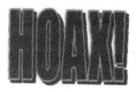

Rx drugs guarantee you will get worse, but you can cure your blood pressure without drugs.

Since healthy blood vessels determine the longevity of every organ in the entire body, you need this book even if you don't have high blood pressure, for vascular health is key to total body health and longevity.

This is the ultimate plan for vascular health.

Sherry A. Rogers, M.D.

Sand Key Company, Inc.
PO Box 40101
Sarasota, FL 34242

The High Blood Pressure Hoax!

Sherry A Rogers, M.D.

Sand Key Company, Inc.
PO Box 40101
Sarasota, FL 34242

1-800-846-6687
www.prestigepublishing.com

Library of Congress Control Number: 2005929036

ISBN: 1-887202-05-6

Printed in the United States of America

Table of Contents

Chapter III: An Oil Change for Your Silver Lining   63

Chapter IV: The Heavy Metal Connection   93

Chapter VII: The Mind and Soul Connection   234

Books By the Author   255
Index   273

Dedication

To Luscious

We come from totally different worlds. To me IBD means irritable bowel disease, to him it's *Investor's Business Daily*. MCI to me is mild cognitive impairment or early Alzheimer's disease, to him it's a telecommunications company. Heavy metals are an investment commodity to him, while to me they are one of the most potent hidden causes of disease. And when I saw him reading a book about hedge funds, I thought we were saving for a gardening project.

We couldn't be any more different. Clearly out of the billions of people in the world, God placed him in mine. How else could this miracle have happened? He makes the Biblical command, "Submit to your husband as to the Lord" easy (*Ephesians* 5:22), for after 36 years, he still continues to grow more luscious every day.

Foreword

The last time I stayed up all night to finish reading a book was over 30 years ago -- I simply had to figure out "who done it" in a thrilling murder mystery that had me engrossed to its very last page. The other night I did it again, but this time it was *The High Blood Pressure Hoax!* that had me spellbound. I don't even have hypertension (yet), but I just couldn't put down this absolutely riveting page-turner.

The High Blood Pressure Hoax! is the latest in a series of inspired and inspiring contributions to the field of environmental medicine by Dr. Sherry Rogers, an extraordinarily gifted and eminently qualified physician whose illustrious career has spanned some 35 years and has enabled her to touch the lives of tens of thousands of individuals. In truth, having devoted her professional life to a passionate pursuit of medical truths, she is one of the few doctors I know who has the guts, the brains, and the heart to say it like it is. She promises, and she delivers -- in this book that is at once both disturbingly eye-opening and profoundly empowering. It is a must-read for all health-conscious laypersons and health-care professionals.

Dr. Rogers details how western medicine and the pharmaceutical industry (both of which focus on masking of symptoms with drugs) actually make the "sick get sicker quicker." She presents rather impressively compelling arguments in favor of detective work that empowers the reader to uncover the real causes of symptoms and reverse them without drugs, restoring optimal wellness, often better than it was before. And benefit extends even to the well person focused on longevity, as the health of the vascular system determines the health of every organ in the body.

An outstandingly accessible, deeply satisfying, powerfully convincing, richly textured, challengingly informative, heavily referenced, and refreshingly heartfelt volume, *The High Blood Pressure Hoax!* quite amazingly reads like an exciting murder mystery. Yet because every page is chock full of clinical pearls of medical wisdom and cutting-edge treatment protocols, it is destined to become a classic in medicine and to find its way, eventually, onto everyone's library shelf.

Dr. Sherry Rogers brings a whole new level of sophistication and understanding to the enormously important and complex field of heart disease -- one of the leading causes of murder in the US today. Although certainly sobering because it speaks to something that is a matter of life or death, *The High Blood Pressure Hoax!* is ultimately a story about survival and hope, hope for all those millions and millions suffering from cardiovascular disease -- sometimes an obvious villain in the piece but more often a silent stalker. What is the identity of the real killer? Who really did it? When you read Dr. Rogers' book from beginning to end, you'll find out...

Martha Stark, MD
Faculty, Harvard Medical School
Faculty, Massachusetts Institute for Psychoanalysis
Author, *Working with Resistance,* and *Modes of Therapeutic Action* (Aronson)

About the Author

Sherry A. Rogers, M.D. is a Diplomate of the American Board of Family Practice, Diplomate of the American Board of Environmental Medicine, Fellow of the American College of Allergy, Asthma and Immunology and a Fellow of the American College of Nutrition. She has been in solo private practice in environmental medicine for over a 35 years in Syracuse, NY where she sees patients from all over the world. She has lectured at Oxford and in 6 countries where she has taught well over 100 physician courses, has published over a dozen books including the landmark book *Detoxify or Die* (prestigepublishing.com), 20 scientific papers, textbook chapters on medical journal editorial boards, was environmental medicine editor for *Internal Medicine World Report*, has a referenced newsletter for 16 years, a non-patient consulting service, a lay and professional lecture service, is the guest on over 100 radio shows a year, and more.

Introduction

Everyone should read this book. Yes, even if you do not have high blood pressure. The reasons are many.

(1) First of all the health of every single cell of your body depends on the health of your blood vessels that supply them. If you don't want to get Alzheimer's, then you need a healthy brain, but it is only as healthy as its blood supply. Likewise, if you don't want cancer (or you are trying to heal it), it starts (and spreads) in areas of poor circulation. Even seemingly non-threatening conditions from impotence and dwindling intellect to rosacea and Raynaud's begin with diseased blood vessels, called vasculitis.

(2) Second, this book will show you the dangers of taking prescription medications for every ailment, treating it as though high blood pressure was a deficiency of anti-hypertensive drugs.

(3) Third, it will show you that for every ailment even one as simple as high blood pressure, there are multiple causes and multiple cures. You have a lot to choose from. In fact I would suggest you read the entire book before you chose your program, then carefully reread and study the sections you plan on doing. For by understanding how the litany of causes work, you (who know your body and medical history better than anyone else) have the optimum opportunity for choosing the best solution for you.

I can't wait to empower you! So let's get started.

Chapter 1

High Blood Pressure Medications
Are Down-Right Dangerous

At a relaxing dinner with another couple? One of you has or will shortly have high blood pressure. Look around the bridge table, a golf four-some or a tennis doubles court; chances are **one in four has high blood pressure** (*Chobanian*). And if you are over 60, the odds are that one in two has high blood pressure. Over 68 million Americans have high blood pressure.

High Blood Pressure Is Epidemic

Are you part of the high blood pressure epidemic? If you think not, high blood pressure is even more epidemic than one in four, because docs who are not up-to-date currently define it as a pressure over 140/90. But you will learn this cut-off is wrong and too high for healthful longevity. In fact a new category of high blood pressure has emerged because of this new information. Folks with a systolic blood pressure (the top number) between 140 and 120 systolic are labeled pre-hypertensive, and have higher hospital admissions and earlier deaths (*Russell*). If using the wrong cut-off were not bad enough, a third of the people with high blood pressure do not even know they have it, while over half of the rest do not have a normal blood pressure even though they are on prescribed medications (*Chobanian*).

Why all the fuss? Because high blood pressure triples your chance of early death. And high blood pressure not only (1) triples your chance of early death, but it (2) triples your chance of developing heart failure (which is on average fatal within five years after diagnosis), (3) or a life-long debilitating or often fatal stroke, (4) and coronary artery disease which leads to sudden and fatal heart attack.

In fact, **53% of deaths from all causes are in part due to high blood pressure.** And high blood pressure is not limited to premature heart and brain death, but damages every other organ from kidneys to eyes. You see, high blood pressure is really a disease of the blood vessels, and since blood vessels supply oxygen and nutrition to every organ of the body, any damage to your vessels eventually leads to damage of any organ. In fact, over a third of folks who lose their brain function through Alzheimer's disease or dementia do so because the vessels to the brain were not healthy (*Papademetriou*). And hypertension quadruples your risk of brain rot, since one of its mechanisms is demyelinization, or loss of the actual covering of nerves leaving them functionless.

Sometimes when I'm standing in line at the store, I look down at the legs of men in shorts and sandals. It's like having x-ray vision combined with a blood pressure cuff because I feel like I can see right into their blood vessels. If they have hairless legs, it's not because they shave. That's a sign of poor vascular supply to the skin of the legs. Likewise, little scabs or lesions that look like pimples or insect bites, broken out areas of scattered redness or rashes, ulcers, seborrheic dermatoses (old age spots, sun spots), spider veins or broken blood vessels are also a sign of a diseased vascular system. As well, thickened or discolored toenails show that the vessels are not letting enough nutrients through to kill fungus. I feel like I have a bird's eye view right into their coronary vessels!

This brings us to another important fact for you. Half of the people who suddenly die do not have high blood pressure, high cholesterol or other known risk factors. But they all do have one thing in common, damaged blood vessels. For **damaged blood vessels underlie all diseases,** whether it is obvious high blood pressure or angina from coronary artery plaque or spasm, heart failure, arrhythmia, high cholesterol, leg pain on exercise (claudication), or ruptured aneurysm, or any other disease like cancer, arthritis, diabetes, depression, allergies, fatigue, fibromyalgia, Alzheimer's, Raynaud's, Parkinson's, colitis and more. For the label you get for a disease is garbage you don't need. What you do need to permanently cure a disease without drugs is to know what caused it, not its fabricated name.

Step I for Curing Your Hypertension

First, it goes without saying that if you have high blood pressure you should buy a blood pressure cuff (sphygmomanometer) plus a stethoscope. Any neighbor-hood nurse, school nurse, your doctor's office nurse, local EMT, volunteers, ambulance and firehouse workers can teach you how to use it. High blood pressure treatment classically begins at a level over 145 on the top (systolic but pressure) and 90 on the bottom (diastolic). But research now shows that the best pressure for healthful longevity is 115-125/70-80(*Lancet 335: 10 92-94, 1990, Chobanian, Stamler*). So if you are 120/75 without medications or any of the abnormal tests you will learn about, that is great.

But be careful if you are over 70 years of age, for having a pressure of 110/70 can be a risk for poor brain circulation and early Alzheimer's (*Verghese*). It depends on the rest of

3

your body health or total package. If you already have too much hardening of your arteries, you may be stuck for now with requiring a little higher pressure in order to get adequate perfusion or blood supply to your brain.

And if you already have high blood pressure, you want to know where you're starting from and to be able to monitor it as it starts coming down through natural means that you will learn about here. For example, after your pressure reaches the "standard" cut off of 145/90, you want to notify your doctor that you will need a reduction in your medication as your healing proceeds and your pressure goes lower via your addition natural cures. Otherwise you will feel awful as the pressure goes too low to give you enough circulation to the brain and other organs.

Once you get really proficient at measuring blood pressure in the crease of the elbow (first feeling for and then listening to the brachial artery pulse), you will also want to learn how to measure it at the ankle. Put your stethoscope just below the inside anklebone (at about 5:00 o'clock position on the right one) and the cuff around the calf. Ideally the two pressures should be the same. As the difference between them widens, this is more evidence of arteriosclerosis and narrowing of vessels in the legs, which eventually can cause claudication or pain on stairs and inclines. But more on this later.

HCT Rx for High Blood Pressure Is the Kiss of Death

As soon as somebody gets high blood pressure they are advised to eat an unpalatable low-salt diet and lose weight. When that fails, as it often does, because it is not a universal

4

cure, the first medication prescribed is a fluid pill to reduce the volume and pressure in the blood vessels. It is simple plumbing. Lowering the amount of fluid flowing through the pipes lowers the pressure, hence medicine's first drug of choice is a diuretic, usually hydrochlorothiazide or HCT. Unfortunately diuretics have many side effects that negate their usefulness. In fact they guarantee earlier death.

First of all, diuretics cause a silent loss of potassium. But for some folks, *an improperly diagnosed potassium deficiency (more on that later) is often the underlying cause of the high blood pressure to begin with. Taking a medication that silently lowers potassium even further leads to higher blood pressure and guarantees the need for stronger medications* in a few years. Meanwhile, low potassium causes palpitations and cardiac arrhythmias that require even more medications. As well, low potassium makes people irritable, tired, and weak, as just a few of the symptoms. Conversely, taking potassium or going on a high potassium diet as you will learn, has corrected hypertension (*Krishna, Valdes, Cappuccio*).

So you can properly categorize your medication, the names of some of the more common diuretics include HCT (hydrochlorthiazide), Aldactone, Aldactazide (spironolactone with HCT), Bumex, Diuril (chlorthiazide), Dyrenium, Enduron, Edecrin, Lasix, Lozol, Maxzide, Midamor, Moduretic, Zaroxolyn, and more. It is easy to ask your cardiologist what class of drug you are on, and whether it contains a diuretic.
If potassium loss were not enough, diuretics also cause the loss of magnesium. But for many people their *high blood pressure is caused by a deficiency of magnesium* in the first place (more on this later). So if you were one of the many whose high blood pressure started because they were low in mag-

nesium, taking a drug that silently lowers it further guarantees you will need even more medicines as the diuretic flushes out more magnesium every day and your pressure climbs higher. As magnesium deficiency silently increases, other symptoms are triggered by it, including mysterious back spasms that are often blamed on old disc injuries, muscle spasms, migraines, spastic colon, eye twitches, asthma, depression, insomnia, heart arrhythmias, Raynaud's, or angina. And undiagnosed magnesium deficiency that continues to be untreated eventually can lead to a sudden heart attack with instant death (*Siskovick, Warram*).

You probably think as I did that most docs will check for magnesium. Wrong. When researchers looked at folks dying in the hospital of various heart problems, well over half of them were low in magnesium. But guess what? A study published in the *Journal of the American Medical Association* showed that **9 out of 10 doctors taking care of these hospitalized patients never looked at their magnesium before they died** (*Whang*). They never thought of testing it, even though it contributed to their untimely death. Now this study of incompetent docs did not take place in East Podunk, but in the sophisticated medical mecca of Boston. In addition, if they had lived, undiagnosed magnesium deficiency can lead to Alzheimer's disease, hypertension, cardiac arrhythmia and sudden heart attack (*Rogers*). This is but one example of the domino effect that occurs when you take drugs, for a drug taken for one disease or symptom can lead quickly to many other symptoms and then further drugs. It becomes a vicious cycle, which inevitably leads to earlier death.

So how did diuretics become the mainstay for the first-line treatment of high blood pressure? Certainly high blood pressure isn't a deficiency of diuretics! It turns out there is an "authoritative" set of guidelines for all physicians to follow. This directive for treating all diseases is called the practice guidelines. And when you look at the recipe for any disease, they practically all come out as a deficiency of some drug. You have arthritis? Take a drug. High cholesterol? Take a drug. How did medicine ever get reduced to a level where every symptom becomes a deficiency of the latest drug? Well scientists looked as the panel of "experts" who create the rules, the practice guidelines, and found that over 87% of these "experts" were financially linked to the pharmaceutical industry (*Choudhry, New England Journal of Medicine, Feb. 2002*)! The "experts" are on the payroll of the drug industry. How's that for what polite folks refer to as misguided medicine?

Protect Yourself with the Right Tests

Would it surprise you to know that the practice guidelines do not require or even mention that a physician check your RBC (red blood cell) potassium and RBC magnesium *before* putting you on a diuretic to see if these deficiencies are causing your high blood pressure in the first place? Nor do they require or even suggest that the RBC levels be checked after you have been on a medication, even for years! Pay close attention here, for if a doctor merely checks the serum levels (which are the standard test), these are worthless because they're too insensitive. You must get **RBC** (red blood cell or erythrocyte) magnesium and potassium, or better yet a whole mineral panel that includes many more minerals, which I will tell you more about later.

7

How can you begin to protect yourself from inferior pharmaceutical-dictated medicine? If your doctor orders potassium and magnesium from a regular local lab, be sure to get a copy of your lab report to determine if he has done the correct test. If it merely says potassium or magnesium, it is wrong. It must say RBC (red blood cell) or erythrocyte potassium and RBC or erythrocyte magnesium. The reason? Potassium and magnesium are not floating around aimlessly in the serum or plasma with nothing to do. Their higher and more important levels are inside the cell, so that's where you have to look for them.

Less than 1% of the magnesium for the entire body is in the serum. That's why the serum magnesium (the wrong serum blood test may also just say "magnesium", and may not even say serum or plasma) can look totally normal even though your magnesium is so low you can have a fatal heart attack within five minutes. No wonder there is a higher rate of fatal heart attack in folks taking diuretics (*Warram*). Likewise the potassium concentration inside the cell is 150 mEq/L and outside the cell 3.5-5.0 mEq/L (*Oh*). So where would you measure it to get the most sensitive and accurate measure? Inside the cell. Unfortunately, the norm is to order it outside the cell, serum potassium, and the one that hides abnormally low potassium indefinitely (*Oh*).

So without checking your RBC minerals, bare minimum, you have not had even the most rudimentary work-up for finding some of the most commonly curable causes for hypertension. And what's even more tragic is **the very medicines that are routinely recommended and prescribed for the treatment of hypertension guarantee that your hypertension will get worse.** For diuretics notoriously lower both minerals. The very top recommended prescribed medicines guarantee that you'll need more medications. For example, you may get a fatal cardiac arrhythmia requiring more medications or a pacemaker from the undiagnosed mineral deficiencies, if you don't get sudden cardiac death first. But as the February 2002 *New England Journal of Medicine* showed us, over 87% of the practice guidelines are made by physicians who are on the payroll of the pharmaceutical companies. So what more can we expect than for every symptom to turn out to be a deficiency of some drug?

HCT Guarantees Heart and Brain Disease

If driving the potassium and magnesium out of the body were not enough reason to avoid taking hydrochlorothiazide (HCT) or any diuretic for high blood pressure, consider this. **Hydrochlorothiazide actually raises the homocysteine level 16%** (*Westphal*). And homocysteine causes high blood pressure (*Kuan*). So you are guaranteed to worsen, requiring even more medications with dangerous side effects.

Homocysteine is one of the crystal ball tests that has been known for decades and should be a part of every smart physical. For it is an amino acid in the bloodstream of humans that is in high amounts in those who are destined to have early heart attacks, Alzheimer's, stroke, schizophrenia, depression, cancer, infertility, chronic pain, hypothyroidism, diabetes, Parkinson's, colitis, macular degeneration (major cause of adult blindness), cataracts, chemical sensitivity, high blood pressure and other degenerative diseases along with accelerated aging (*Braly, Chen*).

9

In fact, when you have hypertension, part of the work-up should automatically include a homocysteine level to make sure that you're not at even greater coronary risk than you already are with just high blood pressure. For homocysteine is one of the many crystal ball tests that alerts docs to know that you have some special risks for earlier disease than most folks. The good news is that when you find elevated homocysteine, you can also find the cause and completely fix it. So you don't have to die an early death from it after all. More on this later, for luckily there are many things that can return the level to normal.

Luckily, by reducing your homocysteine you lower your risk of heart death 50%, lower your chance of cancer death 26%, and death from other diseases including strokes by 104%. So you have to be nuts to prescribe HCT without at least checking the intracellular potassium and magnesium as well as the homocysteine. And if it was missed initially, these three definitely should be checked if you are on diuretics. If you have not at least had these tests, ask your doctor to order the **RBC Minerals** (includes RBC potassium and RBC magnesium as well as other important minerals) and a **Cardiovascular Risk Panel** (both from MetaMetrix) which includes homocysteine and many other crucial markers for early heart attacks. More on these tests later.

The bottom line is **hydrochlorothiazide, the number one recommended treatment for hypertension, dangerously lowers your potassium, magnesium, and other nutrients while raising your risk of heart attack and stroke by raising the homocysteine levels.** *It has over three mechanisms to make you worse and accelerate your disease and aging.* What a deal! So check your lab data and be sure you have at least had **RBC Minerals** and a **Cardiovascular Risk Panel** that includes homocysteine. If you have not had these rudimentary basics, you may want to search for a new doctor.

And one more nasty trick the pharmaceutical/medical alliance pulls on innocent people. When hydrochlorothiazide fails to control your blood pressure, which it inevitably will since you have to get worse as you lose more potassium and magnesium, the next most commonly prescribed drug is often from a category called calcium channel blockers, a leader being Norvasc® (more on these later). Once prescribed, these are usually needed for life, since many docs fail to show you how to find the causes and cures that could make it so you no longer need medications.

Calcium Channel Blockers Shrink the Brain

You'll never guess what one of the side effects of these calcium channel blockers is. They are proven by MRI (magnetic resonance imaging, a sophisticated type of x-ray or brain scan) to cause **shrinking of the brain within five years** (*Archives of Internal Medicine*). And along with this brain shrinking away from the skull, there is gradual loss of intellect, decision-making, reflexes, memory, personality, emotional control and much more (*Psaty, Fitzpatrick, Heckbert*). And calcium channel blockers raise the risk of other diseases like cancer. This is just another example of how the **sick get sicker quicker** when they take drugs, instead of finding and fixing the underlying actual causes of symptoms. If these docs knew enough molecular biochemistry, they would know that magnesium is nature's calcium channel blocker, but more on that later. I will show you how to heal the calcium channels as well (*Iseri*).

11

No wonder that a Professor of Public Health Science at Wake Forest University School of Medicine, Winston-Salem, NC, spoke out so fervently against calcium channel blockers at the 22nd European Society of Cardiology Annual Congress in Amsterdam (*Susman*). Patients taking CCBs (calcium channel blockers) have an over 26% increase in risk of having a heart attack and/or heart failure on these drugs. Furthermore, they are useless, providing less than 0.1 mm Hg reduction in blood pressure compared with other classes of blood pressure drugs. This is not a typo. This means that with the normal blood pressure cuff you cannot even measure the difference of improvement, because it is so small. "This minimal difference is statistically and clinically insignificant" he is quoted to say. His conclusions are that CCBs are expensive, useless and a blatant danger. I couldn't agree more, and he didn't mention their shrinking the brain. Common names of CCBs include Adalat, Cardene, Cardizem, Covera, DynaCirc, Isoptin, Nimotop, Plendil, Procardia, Sular, Tiazac, Verelan, Norvasc, and more continually emerge.

Calcium Channel Blockers Also Promote Cancer

And don't think that you can get off that easily with only an increased rate of heart attack and senility with CCBs. They also increase the rate of cancer, as they should if they represent such enormous abnormality of the cell membrane (*Fitzpatrick*). For think about it. If the cell membrane is damaged enough to need CCBs to stop all the pores from admitting calcium, then the vast majority of calcium channels are shot, dysfunctional. They are so malformed that calcium just surges right into the cell because the membrane gates in the channels are all destroyed. This means that more than just the pores are destroyed. Because the channels are so numerous and close together (the microscopic repeating distance of calcium channels on the cell surface is four times the channel diameter), this means the whole membrane itself is shot in many other ways. More on how to totally repair this later.

Likewise, if the cell membrane is destroyed, then the cell surface gap junctional proteins (or connexins) are also destroyed. These are like little microscopic tubules that connect one cell to another, like a phone line. In this way cells communicate with each other and it is one of the ways that cell growth is regulated. For a cell can shout down the line in the liver, for example, and say, "Hey, you cells down at the end. Yeah, you guys. Stop growing. You are crowding us out up here." But pesticides and other environmental chemicals rip these gap junctional proteins or tubules off the surface of cell membranes. Now that the phone lines are cut, cells can no longer communicate. One result? Unregulated growth, which we call cancer. Another result from such damaged cell membranes is high blood pressure.

Wild unrestricted growth without concern for neighboring cells can be tamed by many nutrients that cause the regrowth of these tubules. In fact that is how high doses of vitamin A reverse some types of leukemia. They restore the phone lines or communication tubules (connexins) to the surfaces of cells so they can now communicate again with other cells and tell them to stop wildly growing as though they were cancer cells (more details for those who want them in *Wellness Against All Odds*).

You can now understand why CCBs are particularly dangerous to be taking if you already have cancer. For the cancer cell contains only 1% of the calcium of a normal cell. That is one of the biochemical abnormalities that fuel wild cancer growth and metastases. So taking a CCB lowers the calcium even further in the cancer cell by blocking entry, thus further disturbing normal chemistry.

Magnesium Is Nature's CCB

And how do you repair the membrane? By restoring the sandwich layers of fatty acids that have become depleted by years of wrong diets, which we will explore in the trans fatty acid section in Chapter III. Meanwhile, wouldn't it be wonderful if there were something natural, inexpensive, readily available and terribly safe that would substitute for a calcium channel blocker? Well there is. Magnesium is nature's calcium channel blocker (*Iseri*). But some membranes are so badly damaged over the years that they need more than just restoration of the magnesium. They need an oil change, which you'll learn about in Chapter III. And as you will learn, stress also triggers high blood pressure, but enough magnesium can negate that in many ways (*Kh*).

Diuretics Also Trigger Diabetes

Studies show that folks who treat their blood pressure with diuretics, beta-blockers and/or hydralazine, other common classes of drugs, get much more diabetes (*Skarfors*). And you can understand why they developed another disease, since they never fixed the causes of the first one. These studies show that over 10 years, not only do they develop diabetes, but they get high triglycerides as well. So they now have two diseases that hasten cardiovascular death, caused by

14

taking a drug that is supposed to prevent death by lowering one cardiovascular parameter, the blood pressure.

The scary part is that papers showing these drugs trigger diabetes go back as far as over 30 years ago and are still being published, yet ignored (*Breckenridge, Ames, Tanaka, Waal-Manning, Day*). Incredible, the power of the pharmaceutical industry to get physicians so enamored by drugs that they bypass basic medical research (*Angell, Cohen, Haley*). History has shown that if this were a vitamin that caused all these problems, it would be off the market in a flash.

Another worrisome category of blood pressure drugs, called *ACE inhibitors*, actually increases the risk of anaphylaxis (serious and potentially fatal allergic reaction) as much as 20 fold higher than normal (*Kemp*). And a particularly sneaky side effect of ACE inhibitors is *chronic cough* that no one can figure out. Some of the 27 medications that are ACE (or angiotensin converting enzyme) inhibitors include such names as Accupril, Altace, Captopril, Lotensin, Monopril, Prinivil, Univasc, Vasotec, Zestril, Accuretic (an ACE inhibitor with the diuretic, hydrochlothiazide), Aceon, Atacand, Avalide (also contains a diuretic), Avapro, Capoten, Capozide (also with a diuretic), Cozaar, Diovan, and more. A veritable alphabet soup! They, like all drugs, have whole pages of side effects in the book of drugs, PDR (*Physician's Desk Reference*).

Did you notice that these last two categories of drugs are blockers and inhibitors? This is a recurring theme among drugs. When a pathway is malfunctioning, rather than step in and find a simple deficiency and correct it, a drug is prescribed for a lifetime that turns off or blocks the malfunctioning chemistry. Sort of like driving down the highway in your car and upon seeing the red oil light go on, smashing it with a hammer. This is analogous to taking a drug, for you have solved the problem of the irritating warning light. But since you haven't fixed the problem, you are inevitably headed for disaster.

There are other categories of anti-hypertensive drugs that work on the nervous system. For there are tiny nerves wrapped around blood vessels that control how tightly the blood vessel muscles squeeze. The tighter they are the higher the pressure. These include Aldomet (generic methyldopa) or Aldoril (methyldopa plus a diuretic), Apresaline (hydralazine), Cardura, Catapres, and more.

And I hesitate to tell you more bad news about drugs (which would actually fill volumes), but remember the Vioxx® (generic name rofecoxib) scam? Merck's billion-dollar blockbuster pain and arthritis medicine that was supposed to spare the stomach from ulcers but didn't. Worse yet, they found that it could quadruple your risk of sudden death from clots (*Fitzgerald*). For example, one beautiful woman in her early 30s who was in great shape with no heart disease died of a sudden heart attack within a month of starting it. And **prestigious journals warned of this side effect every year for FIVE years,** (as did I in *TW*), while the FDA ignored these researchers from the top medical schools (*Fitzgerald, Topol*). This is the lobbying power of billion dollar drugs.

Well that is not the end of the story. **Vioxx also causes high blood pressure** (*Fitzgerald*). In fact many of the NSAID (non-steroidal anti-inflammatory drugs, like ibuprofen, Motrin, Naprosyn, Celebrex, etc.) painkillers raise blood pressure (*Mathews*). But who is suspicious of their knee medicine when they develop high blood pressure? They just think it came out of the blue like all diseases of aging. And when you do make the association and then go to the expense of proving it, it is conveniently ignored. Most other NSAIDs related to it, like Bextra (also removed) do the same thing.

The Magnesium Miracle May Solve Your Hypertension

So what is the first step? Since government studies show that the average American diet only provides 40%, or less than half the magnesium a person needs in a day, you can understand why there is such an epidemic of high blood pressure. The world's expert who has been studying magnesium for over half a century reports that 80% of the population is deficient, which certainly compliments what I have observed over 35 years (*Seelig*). On the flip side, studies confirm that the greater the intake of magnesium, the lower one's risk of developing heart disease, sudden death, and high blood pressure. No wonder post mortem analyses of hearts of folks unlucky enough to die of a heart attack show the hearts to be 22% lower than normal in magnesium and potassium (*Johnson*). No question, **diuretics kill, partly by causing earlier heart attacks** (*Warram, Siscovick*).

For many folks all they need to do is increase their daily magnesium to 400-600 mg and they won't even have high blood pressure (*Itoh, Motoyama, Widman*). This is easy to do with **Natural Calm** (Peter Gillham's) one tsp. 1-3 times a day in a glass of water or **Magnesium Chloride Solution 85 mg/cc** (Pain & Stress Center), 1-2 cc 3-4 times a day. Or perhaps you're lucky enough to have a physician who reads *TW* (*Total Wellness*, my monthly subscription newsletter for 16

years, designed to keep folks up on the latest information).
Then he knows about the most potent form of prescription
magnesium and can write a prescription for you for **Magnesium Chloride Solution 200 mg/cc** (Windham Pharmacy,
see Dec. 2003 *TW* for prescribing details). **You want at least
400-600 mg of magnesium a day.**

The best way to correct potassium is with the whole foods
diet along with carrot juicing, but more on that as well as reducing your homocysteine later. And I'll map out a plan for
your laboratory tests, diet and nutrients later. Right now I
want you to get a handle on how dangerously deceptive the
current treatment of hypertension is.

Bare minimum for testing you want **RBC Minerals** (Meta-
Metrix), which includes both RBC potassium and RBC magnesium. But hold off just yet, for I'm going to show you how
to cover even more curable causes of your high blood pressure and vascular disease and how to save you money on
laboratory tests at the same time. Meanwhile, I hope I've
made it clear that without the information on these tests,
your doctor is working blindly and missing out on finding
some very rudimentary and easily remedied causes of hypertension and hidden vascular disease, not to mention
missing out on optimally keeping you alive. For recall as I
intimated in the beginning, even if you don't have high
blood pressure yet, many other diseases begin with hidden
vascular disease or vascular dysfunction. You may have silent vascular inflammation that produces no symptoms yet,
as you will learn in the next chapter. So what you will learn
here has a great chance of healing lots more than just hypertension. In fact vascular health is fundamental for healing

any condition and for retarding aging and promoting youthful longevity as well as the sports' advantage.

Consider this: the *Journal of the American Medical Association* shows that more than a quarter of a million people die each year just from medical errors, over 12,000 from unnecessary surgery, over 80,000 from hospital-acquired infections, and over 106,000 die in the hospital from drug reactions, that are recognized and admitted to (*Lazarou*). This makes drug reactions the 3rd cause of death! But this doesn't count the insanity that you are about to learn here. In fact this doesn't even count those who die outside of the hospital or those for whom the real cause of death was not appreciated. Clearly the mainstay of "modern" medical treatment is a drug that merely covers up symptoms by poisoning enzymes. This allows the process to worsen as it is simultaneously accelerated by the side effects of drugs. As well, many Harvard and other specialists have written extensively about the hazards of drug-oriented medicine (*Glenmullen, Breggin, Moore, Epstein, Fagin, Moss, Cohen, Angell*). After reading all these you can appreciate that **medical treatment with drugs is actually the number one cause of death.**

The good news is that you can painlessly learn how to prevent all this. So get going on some magnesium and let's get started on the rest of your journey toward becoming independently healthy.

Crystal Ball Test for Fatal Heart Disease

Go to the greatest cardiologist in the country and ask him for the best test that shows your chances of dying early from a heart attack. Two to one he will use your cholesterol level and your blood pressure as indicators, since these are part of the standard that physicians follow (because there are drugs for them). But as it turns out, numerous studies show that elevated cholesterol levels have practically no bearing on early heart attacks or strokes. Blood pressure is a little better, but still is far outperformed by a crystal ball test that is far superior, your Vitamin E level. And if you add the vitamins A and C levels to it, you improve the crystal ball prognostic ability more than 21% beyond to a total of 90% probability (*Gey*). Wow! **Knowing your vitamins A, C and E levels give you a 90% accurate forecast of your chances of early heart death.** An *ACE* in the hole (pardon the pun, I couldn't control myself) if I ever saw one.

But because medicine is owned by the pharmaceutical industry, we merely check for parameters like cholesterol and blood pressure, for which there are drugs you can take until the day you die. And of course, that day comes sooner since the blood pressure drugs for hypertension, for example, are draining you of magnesium and potassium while raising your homocysteine level and shrinking your brain.

The current standard in medicine is to work blindly and fail to check your nutrient levels with an **ION Panel** (which includes among other life-saving tests, indicators of whether you have sufficient life-saving vitamins A, C, and E). I have no other premise but to assume it is because those deficiencies could be repaired easily and quickly with nutrients. Worse yet for the pharmaceutical industry, once you have corrected sufficient deficiencies, you may not even need lifelong medications, because correcting the ACE deficiencies could, in some folks, also correct their hypertension, cholesterol metabolism and other ailments. A further beauty of knowing your nutrient levels is that by correcting them you will forestall numerous other symptoms and diseases that would have eventually emerged. Given the financial and bureaucratic pressures in medicine, it may not be in our lifetimes when measuring nutrients becomes standard. It's up to you to get yours now and to take nutrients that keep you in the higher percentile. For now, why not start with A, C, E, in the form of **ACES** (vitamins A, C, E, plus selenium), one a day for insurance. This is your ACE in the hole.

My recommendations? At least yearly get an **ION Panel** (by MetaMetrix) that includes your RBC minerals plus vitamins A, C, E and much more at 50% savings when you roll so many important tests into one panel. I'll tell you more later. In the meantime at least take something as simple and easy as one or two of Carlson's **ACES** daily, which contains 5000 units of beta-carotene (that transforms into vitamin A), 500 mg of vitamin C, 200 units of vitamin E (d-alpha-tocopherol), 50 mcg of selenium as well as the additional carotenoids alpha-carotene, cryptoxanthinm zeaxanthin and lutein. You can easily add this to your daily multiple because your need for extra antioxidants is forever increasing. I prefer their **ACES with Zinc**, which adds zinc, crucial in keeping your genetics from becoming damaged by environmental chemicals and triggering cancer, and also needed as I will show for your vessel health.

Aging Begins with Mr. ED

Even if you are healthy, experts agree, aging begins in the vascular tree (*Celermajer*), so let's roll over to Chapter II to learn what goes on inside your blood vessels.

Product Sources:

- Natural Calm, Peter Gillham, 1-888-800-1180
- Magnesium Citrate 166 mg (Metabolic Maintenance) Pain & Stress Center, or Magnesium Chloride 85 mg/cc, Pain & Stress Center, 1-800-669-CALM
- Magnesium Chloride Solution 200 mg/cc, Rx needed, Windham Pharmacy, 1-518-734-3033
- ACES with Zinc, carlsonlabs.com, 1-800-323-4141
- RBC Minerals, MetaMetrix, 1-800-221-4640
- ION Panel (includes above), metametrix.com, 1-800-221-4640
- Cardiovascular Risk Panel, MetaMetrix, 1-800-221-4640

(Magnesium choices take 400-600 mg a day)

N.E.E.D.S. (often referred to as NEEDS) is a mail order company that has been supplying our patients and readers for over 2 decades with most of the nutrients you will find recommended in the Product Sources at the end of every chapter, 1-800-634-1380.

References:

Note that the tiny names you find in parentheses through the text of this book are the authors of just some of the scientific studies that support what I have told you. Even more references are included in the reference sections following each chapter. I did not put the back-up in parentheses after every fact because it makes reading too clumsy. But in the reference sections you will find the backup for everything in the text. This scientific backup is particularly important for your doctor, to bring him/her into the 21st century of medicine. For we now have the tools from environmental, nutritional and molecular biochemistry with which to find the causes and cures of symptoms, not just blindly drug every symptom and lead folks into a cascading use of side effect-laden drugs. Because the pharmaceutical industry has such control over medical education, most of this is not yet taught in medical schools, even though all this research comes from some of the most brilliant minds on medical school faculties. Hence, I need to arm you with the evidence that will protect you from the undereducated.

A book on homocysteine I recommend is *The H Factor Solution* by J Braly and P Holford, Basic Health Public, N. Bergen NJ, 1-201-868-8336

Chobanian ABV, et al, The 7th report of the Joint National Committee on Prevention, Detection, Evaluation and Treatment of High Blood Pressure: the JNC 7 report, *J Am Med Assoc*, 289: 2560-72, 2003

Stamler J, Stamler R, Neaton JD, et al, Low risk factor profile and long-term cardiovascular and noncardiovascular mortality and life expectancy: findings for five large cohorts of young adult and middle-aged men and women, *J Am Med Assoc*, 282; 21:2012-18, Dec 1, 1999

Verghese J, et al, Low blood pressure and risk of dementia in very old individuals, *Neurol*, 61; 12: 1667-72, 2003

Westphal S, Rading A, Luley C, Dierkes J, Antihypertensive treatment and homocysteine concentrations, *Metabolism*, 52; 3:261-3, Mar. 2003

Abbott RD, et al, Dietary magnesium intake and the future risk of coronary heart disease (the Honolulu Heart Program). *Am J Cardiol*, 92; 6: 665-69, Sept. 15, 2003

Starfield B, Is US health really the best in the world? *J Amer Med Assoc* 284; 4:483-5, July 26, 2000

Lazarou J, Pomeranz BH, Corey PN, Incidence of adverse drug reactions in hospitalized patients, *J Amer Med Assoc*, 279; 15:1200-1205, Apr. 15, 1998

Seeliig CB, Magnesium deficiency in hypertension uncovered by magnesium load retention, *J Amer Clin Nutr* 8; 5:455, abs. 113, 1989

Mountokalakis, Diuretic-induced magnesium deficiency, *Magnesium* 2:57, 1983

Altura BM, Altura BT, New perspectives on the role of magnesium in the pathophysiology of cardiovascular system, II. Experimental; aspects, *Magnesium* 4:245-71, 1985

Singh RB, Cameron EA, Relation of myocardial magnesium deficiency to sudden death in ischaemic heart disease, *Amer Heart J*, 103; 3:399-450, 1982

Psaty BM, Heckbert SR, Furberg CD, et al, The risk of myocardial infarction associated with antihypertensive drug therapies, *J Amer Med Assoc*, 1995; 274:620-625

Fitzpatrick AL, Daling JR, Weissfeld JL, et al, Use of calcium channel blockers and breast carcinoma risk in postmenopausal women, *Cancer*, 1997; 80:1438-1447

Heckbert SR, Longstreth WT, Furberg CD, et al, The association of antihypertensive agents with MRI white matter findings and with modified mini-mental state examination in older adults, *J Amer Geriat Soc* 45:1423-1433, 1997

Iseri LT, French JH, Magnesium: Nature's physiologic calcium blocker, *Amer Heart J*, 108; 1:188-192, 1984

Whang R, Ryder KW, Frequency of hypomagnesemia and hypermagnesemia, requested versus routine, *J Amer Med Assoc*, 263:3063-64, 1990

Rogers SA, *Depression Cured At Last!*, Prestige Publishing, Syracuse NY, 1998 (prestigepublishing.com or 1-800-846-6687)

Krishna G, Gopal MD, Kapoor SC, Potassium depletion exacerbates essential hypertension, *Ann Int Med* 115; 2:77-83, July 15, 1991

Valdes G, et al, Potassium supplementation lowers blood pressure and increases urinary kallikrein in hypertensives, *J Hum Hypert* 5:91-6, 1991

Cappuccio FP, et al, Potassium supplementation for hypertension: A meta-analysis, *J Hypert* 9:465-73, May 1991

Oh MS, Water, Electrolyte, and Acid-base Balance, Chapter 6, p. 127, in Shils, ME, Olson JA, Shike M, eds., *Modern Nutrition*, 8th Ed., 1994, Lea & Febinger, Philadelphia

Johnson CJ, et al, Myocardial tissue concentration of magnesium and potassium in men dying suddenly from ischemic heart disease, *Amer J Clin Nutr* 32:967-70,

Shils ME, Experimental production of magnesium deficiency in man, *Ann NY Acad Sci*, 162:847-855

Warram JH, Lori LMB, Valsania P, Chrislieb AR, Krolewski AS, Excess mortality associated with diuretic therapy in diabetes mellitus, *Arch Intern Med* 151:1350-6, 1991

Siscovick DS, Raghunathan TE, et al, Diuretic therapy for hypertension and the risk of primary cardiac arrest, *N Engl J Med* 330:1852-7, 1994

Seelig M, Cardiovascular consequences of magnesium deficiency and loss: Pathogenesis, prevalence, and manifestations of magnesium and chloride loss in refractory potassium repletion, *Amer J Cardiol* 53, 4g-21g, 1989

Baker SM, Magnesium in primary care and preventive medicine: clinical correlation of magnesium loading studies, *Magnes Tr Elements*, 10:251-62, 1991-1992

Rogers SA, Unrecognized magnesium deficiency masquerades as diverse symptoms: Evaluation of an oral magnesium challenge test, *Internat Clin Nutr Rev* 11; 3:117-125 or 26-30, July 1991

Skarfors ET, Llthell HO,Selinas I, Aberg H, Do antihypertensive drugs precipitate diabetes in predisposed men?, *Brit Med J*, 298: 1147-1152, Apr. 29, 1989

Breckenridge A, Dollery CT, Fraser R, et al, Glucose tolerance in a hypertensive patients on long-term diuretic treatment, *Lancet*,i: 64-4, 1967

Ames RP, Hill P, Increase in serum lipids during treatment of hypertension with chlorthalidone, *Lancet*, i: 721-3, 1976

Tanaka N, Sakaguchi S, Oshige K, Nimura T, Kanehisa T, Effect of chronic administration of propanolol on lipoprotein composition, *Metabolism* 25: 1071-5, 1976

Kemp SF, Lieberman P, Inhibitors of angiotensin II: potential hazards for patients at risk for anaphylaxis, *Ann Allergy* 1997; 78:527-9

Susman E, Class of BP drugs linked to excess deaths, *Internal Medicine World Report*, 15; 10: 1, 8, Sept 1, 2000

Waal-Manning HJ, Simpson FO, Beta-blockers and lipid metabolism, *Brit Med J*, 7: 705,1977

Day JL, Simpson N, Metcalfe J, Page RL, Metabolic consequences of atenolol and propanolol in treatment of essential hypertension, *Brit Med J*, 9: 77-80, 1979

Grossman E, Messerli FH, et al, Does diuretic therapy increase the risk of renal cell carcinoma? *Am J Cardiol*, 83:1090-93, Apr 1, 1999

Angell M, M.D., (former editor of the *New England Journal of Medicine*), *The Truth About Drug Companies*, Random House, NY, 2004

Glenmullen J, *Prozac Backlash*, Simon & Schuster, NY, 2000

Breggin PR, *Talking Back to Ritalin*, Common Courage Press, P.O. Box 702, Munroe ME 04951, 1998

Breggin PR, *Toxic Psychiatry*, St. Martin' s Press, NY, 1991

Moore TJ, *Deadly Medicine*, Simon & Schuster, NY, 1995

Epstein SS, *The Politics of Cancer Revisited*, East Rage Press, Fremont Center, NY, 1998

Haley D, *Politics In Healing, The Suppression and Manipulation of American Medicine*, Potomac Valley Press, Washington D.C., 2000

Fagin D, Lavelle M, Center for Public Integrity, *Toxic Deception. How the chemical industry manipulates science, bends the law, and endangers your health.* A Birch Lane Press, Carol Publishing, 120 Enterprise Ave., Secaucus NJ 07094, 1996

Moss RW, *Questioning Chemotherapy*, Equinox Press, NY, 1995

Moore, TJ *Prescription for Disaster*, Simon & Schuster, NY, 1998

25

Cohen JS, *Over Dose, The Case Against the Drug Companies*, Tarcher/Penguin/Putnam, NY, 2001

Choudhry NK, Stelfox HT, Detsky AS, Relationships between authors of clinical practice guidelines and the pharmaceutical industry, *J Am Med Assoc*, 287; 5:612-617, Feb 6, 2002

Fitzpatrick AL, Daling JR, Weissfeld JL, et al, Use of calcium channel blockers and breast carcinoma risk in postmenopausal women, *Cancer*, 1997; 80:1438-47

Meese S, Hypertension control rates declining, *Internal Med World Rep* 14; 7:1, 36, July 1999

Bankhead C, Cardiovascular drugs could worsen stroke outcome, *Internal Medicine World Report*, 16, May 1999

Kh R, Khullar M, Kashyap M, et al, Effect of oral magnesium supplementation on blood pressure, platelet aggregation and calcium handling in deoxycorticosterone in acetate induced hypertension in rats, *J Hypert*, 18: 9 19-26, 2000

Gey FK, Puska P, Jordan P, Moser UK, Inverse correlation between plasma vitamin E and mortality from ischemic heart disease in cross-cultural epidemiology, *Am J Clin Nutr*, 53:326s-34s, 1991

Celermajer DS, Sorensen KE, Deanfield JE, et al, Aging is associated with endothelial dysfunction in healthy men years before the age-related decline in women, *J Am Coll Cardiol*, 24; 2:471-6, Aug 1994

Itoh K, et al, The effects of high oral magnesium supplementation on blood pressure, serum lipids and related variables in apparently healthy Japanese subjects, *Br J Nutr*, 78; 5:737-50, 1997

Seelig MS, Rosanoff A, *The Magnesium Factor*, NY, Avery Publ, 2003

Motoyama T, et al, Oral magnesium supplementation in patients with essential hypertension, *Hypertension*, 13; 3:227-32, 1989

Widman L, et al, The dose dependent reduction in blood pressure through administration of magnesium. A double-blind placebo-controlled crossover study, *Am J Hypertens*, 6; 141-5, 1993

Kuan YM, Dear EA, Grigg MJ, Homocysteine: and aetiological contributor to peripheral vascular arterial disease, *ANZ J Surg*, 72; 9:668-71, 2002

Chen N, Liu Y, Greiner CD, Holtzman JL, Physiological concentrations of homocysteine inhibit the human plasma GSH peroxidase that reduces organic hydroperoxides, *J Lab Clin Med*, 136; 1:58-65, 2000

Fitzgerald GA, Coxibs and Cardiovascular disease, *New Engl J Med*, 351; 1:1709-11, Oct 21, 2004

Topol EJ, Failing the public health- rofecoxib, Merck, and the FDA, *New Engl J Med*, 351; 1:1707-9, Oct 21, 2004

Russell LB, Valiyeva E, Carson JL, Effects of prehypertension on admissions and deaths, *Arch Intern Med*, 164; 19:2119-24, 2004

Papademetriou V, Blood pressure regulation and cognitive function: A review of the literature, *Geriatrics*, 60;Jan: 20-24, 2005

Mathews AW, Hensley S, FDA conclave will assess cardiac risks of painkillers, *Wall Street J*, B1, B3, Feb. 7, 2005

Dear Reader,

Please note: If sometimes you feel bogged down with chemistry and technicality, remember that (1) you are learning more than most doctors know, (2) there are more choices here than any one person will ever need so you have a fantastic array to chose from, and (3) at the end you will realize in retrospect that you have absorbed and understood more than you ever estimated. In fact, you have now enormously empowered yourself to heal against all odds. So just keep reading. If you find Chapters II, III and IV complicated then skip to Chapter V now and backtrack.

Chapter II

Boost Your Silver Lining of Longevity

Remember the old song, "*Look For the Silver Lining*"? Well you have a silver lining in your body that is a major determinant of how long you will live. We used to think the skin was the largest organ in the body. Peel it off the body spread it out, and it measures a little over a square meter. Then when we began studying the gut and realized that if you spread out all of the fingerlike microscopic villi, the gut was a far larger target organ, comparable in square surface area to more than a tennis court. But there is an organ that we rarely think of that makes even the gut pale in comparison with its enormous size of 6-8 tennis courts. In fact most physicians much less lay people ever give the largest organ in the body a second thought.

The ironic thing is that this organ is only one cell thick, yet it runs through 100,000 miles of blood vessels in your body. It is the *endothelium, the microscopic silver lining to every blood vessel.* You're probably thinking of an average blood vessel that has a muscular layer around it. But when you get right down to the very tiniest capillaries at the end of all major blood vessels, they are only one cell thick. All that remains in capillaries is the endothelial lining. They have no muscular layer like the larger blood vessels.

What's so amazing is that the Master Biochemist of life, God, has engineered a system where the endothelial lining creates a gas that can effortlessly slip through cells to perform its magic. The main function of this cleverly designed gas is to relax blood vessels and stop clots from forming. This *life-*

saving gas is nitric oxide. Dr. Alfred Noble, after whom the Nobel Prize is named, made nitroglycerin explode and later invented dynamite. But he also discovered that nitroglycerin in tiny amounts relaxes the heart blood vessels and relieves angina. In fact, other drugs in common use, like those for erectile dysfunction, Viagra, Levitra and Cialis, also work by boosting the action of nitric oxide (NO). And, you guessed it. What you will learn here about blood pressure you can also use to more safely and inexpensively reverse erectile dysfunction, too.

Meet Mr. ED

No, I'm not talking about the 1970's TV show featuring a talking horse, Mr. ED. I'm introducing you to a new clinical problem that underlies much disease, **endothelial dysfunction.** You see, when the blood vessel lining, the endothelium, is diseased or damaged, it no longer works or functions like it should. It tends to tighten and cause high blood pressure or form clots that lead to heart attacks and strokes. Luckily, NO (nitric oxide gas made in the innermost blood vessel endothelial lining) also heals damaged blood vessels. But when blood vessel walls become loaded down with cholesterol, they don't send out their message to make vessel-expanding (vasodilating) nitric oxide very well.

Many other factors can cause ED, or endothelial dysfunction, like
(1) being several hours after a high fat meal,
(2) being low in various nutrients,
(3) needing an oil change in the cell membranes (which I'll tell you about in the next chapter), and

(4) having too many chemicals like mercury or pesticides stockpiled in the blood vessel lining (Chapter IV). These all contribute to abnormal and impaired endothelial function. And when the blood vessel endothelial lining is not functioning, we don't just get high blood pressure. Every organ in the entire body is in danger of deterioration, dysfunction, and accelerated aging.

But now scientists have discovered how God makes nitric oxide in the endothelial lining. He begins with arginine, a simple amino acid from our foods. In fact researchers have shown that when the blood vessel lining or endothelium is healthy and making enough nitric oxide, this prevents many calamities:
   (1) Nitric oxide relaxes the blood vessel muscles thereby lowering blood pressure,
   (2) it keeps platelets from sticking to the blood vessel wall and forming plaque and occlusions that lead to a heart attack and stroke, and
   (3) it regulates many other enzymes that promote longevity. In fact the endothelium is like a master hormone that talks to all the rest of the body's cells and directs their actions. But most importantly,
   (4) not only does nitric oxide slow plaque growth and
   (5) suppress arteriosclerosis from forming, but
   (6) arginine has *actually melted away plaque that already existed on artery walls.*

This is like the fountain of youth being discovered. There is no medicine that removes plaque from vessels. That's why folks have to resort to angioplasty where cardiologists ream out vessels or bypass surgery where they just give up and replace the old vessels with ones from other parts of the body like the leg, that have not yet become diseased with plaque. Later on I'll show you other nutrients and non-prescription agents that also remove plaque from vessel walls, thereby turning back the hands of time.

ADMA, the Newest and Strongest
Predictor of Heart Death

How fast would you want to do a simple blood test if it could tell you whether you have a quadruple risk of having a heart attack? Especially if the results are totally and easily correctable? You have just learned that a main chemical that our endothelial cells make, those cells that line the inside of blood vessels, is a powerful gas called nitric oxide. Its function is to cause blood vessels to relax and dilate, allowing more blood flow, more precious nutrients and more oxygen to the heart muscle and other tissues. Luckily for us, nitric oxide is made through an enzyme *nitric oxide synthase*. And we can make more of it by adding the simple amino acid **L-arginine** to our diets. In fact L-arginine is such a good vasodilator that it works well for folks with impotence and is considerably cheaper, and safer than the erectile dysfunction drugs that have the ability to cause heart attacks, like Viagra, Levitra or Cialis.

Needless to say we want lots of nitric oxide dilating our vessels. But in *some folks they make too much of a nitric oxide synthase inhibitor called asymmetrical dimethyl arginine*. Translation: They make too much of a protein that turns off normal NO (nitric oxide) formation. They have high levels of a protein that strangles their enzyme that makes NO. Fortunately we can measure this protein that poisons NO with a

31

simple blood test called **ADMA** (asymmetrical dimethyl arginine).

And making too much ADMA causes lots more than just high blood pressure. For when nitric oxide is low because of too much inhibitor, you not only can get high blood pressure, but coronary and carotid (heart and neck arteries) arteriosclerosis, diabetes, cancer, kidney problems, brain problems with loss of good mood and memory loss, arrhythmia, congestive heart failure and much more. In fact in one study, when people were just *at the top of the normal level of ADMA, they had four times the average amount of heart attacks.* And if they were over the top of the normal level for ADMA, they had a 27-fold increased risk of disease (*Valkonen*).

The beauty of this simple blood test is that your doctor can just write on a prescription "**ADMA**". Then you call Meta-Metrix, get the kit, go to any local lab and have the blood drawn. If your levels are high, **L-Arginine Powder**, ½-1 scoop twice a day, is a wonderful first treatment, inexpensive, non-toxic and natural, because it's what nature uses anyway. It reverses the inhibition of nitric oxide and actually causes vasodilatation. As well, arginine is a potent blood thinner, keeping platelets from clumping together abnormally. It has rescued folks with congestive heart failure and improved their blood flow, walking distance without leg pain (claudication) and heart function in general (*Rector*). LDL cholesterol (the bad one, caused in part by trans fatty acids that you will learn about in the next chapter) causes more ADMA to be made. That's one more case where *arginine is useful for slowing down the progression of arteriosclerosis*, especially if someone has high cholesterol or kidney disease (*Zoccali*).

So this is wonderful news. **We know one of the secret causes of accelerated "old age", and it is 100% reversible** if you merely find it first. So be sure you have had the ADMA test done.

Arginine Can Reverse High Blood Pressure

How much arginine does it take to reverse high blood pressure, claudication (pain in legs with walking or on inclines), kidney disease, heart failure, or to keep cholesterol from damaging arteries? The dose that it takes can be pretty high, sometimes as much as 7 grams three times a day. But fortunately when you put a total program together of other complementary nutrients, you can get away with much less. For don't forget researchers never do a full nutritional work-up on these patients to find out their total mineral, fatty acids, vitamin, amino acids, and orphan nutrient deficiencies, nor do they check for their toxicities that need to be removed. The bottom line is folks doing a much more intelligent and biochemically balanced treatment of heart problems can get away with much lower doses and not have to use astronomical doses such as this. Big doses like this come from medical studies where it is often the only thing they treated with. They don't look at the total package of what else is wrong with the person, but they treat a nutrient like a drug.

I would recommend you start with two to four 675 mg **L-Arginine Capsules** (Carlson) twice a day and then check your ADMA (and blood pressure) in a month. Assuming you have looked into many of the things that we will cover here, that may be all you need to do. If you do need higher doses, an excellent trustworthy source, Carlson, makes **L-Arginine Powder**, 4 grams (4000 mg) per teaspoon. Merely dissolve one teaspoon in water twice a day. That is the maximum dose usually needed, so it's fine to start lower and work yourself up slowly. Chances are you won't have to go that high. Your pressure could normalize with ¼ or ½ tsp. twice a day, especially once you get your other nutrients adjusted, as you will learn later. Another option is low dose sustained action **Perfusia-SR** (650 mg).

In the meantime, you guessed it. Lots of other things like smoking and high fat diets, undiagnosed B vitamin deficiencies, trans fatty acids and undiscovered fatty acid deficiencies are just a sampling of the things that inhibit proper nitric oxide synthesis from the endothelial lining. On the flip side, exercise, all sorts of antioxidants I'll tell you about, alkaline water (that increases the antioxidant superoxide dismutase efficiency in the body), cod liver oil, a whole foods diet, your detox cocktail and many other factors promote a healthy endothelium. We will explore them and more together so that you can learn how to healthfully rejuvenate your silver lining, and banish Mr. ED.

Some of you more experienced readers might say that you have heard that taking arginine to boost endothelial function can reactivate old herpes virus and that it does so by lowering the concentration of the amino acid lysine. You may logically wonder if you should be taking lysine with arginine. The answer is no. Since lysine and arginine are taken up by the same transport system in the small intestine, researchers also wondered if taking arginine would inhibit lysine and reactivate latent herpes virus in some folks. However, studies show that there was no difference in lysine levels and concluded that arginine did not interfere with its uptake (*Evans*). In addition, they found that taking nine grams of L-**Arginine Powder** daily (about twice the amount that you get from your diet) had no side effects while it sufficiently increased arginine levels. However it did decrease glycine levels. Since glycine is so necessary to make glutathione (in your detox cocktail) and to help detoxify via other routes, you might as well have it every day anyway, 1-2 **Glycine 500** mg a day.

Two Nutrients Neutralize a High Fat Meal

Imagine. Every time we indulge in a big fat juicy meal, for a couple of hours the NO production is sort of paralyzed. Therefore it is easier for the blood vessels to tighten up and easier for clotting to occur. That is why it is a time of more frequent heart attacks. But as little as 500 mg of vitamin C and 400 IU of vitamin E can rescue us and protect the endothelial lining from spasm and coagulation. So it makes sense to incorporate these two vitamins into your daily armamentarium of nutrients, especially just before bed after your fattest meal of the day (*Plotnick*).

And no wonder studies also show that folks with high blood pressure have extra free radicals in the blood (*Kumar*), have low levels of vitamin E and C, and that higher levels of these nutrients tend to protect folks from hypertension (*Newaz, Duffy, Taddei, Ness*). It all fits and points to the need for getting enough of these two nutrients, C and E, each day.

Let's Get Rid of the Aspirin-Recommending Cardiologists

When a guy goes for a physical and he is over 50, often the cardiologist recommends he take an aspirin a day to decrease his coagulability or clotting ability of the blood and the ability of these clots to cling to the inside of vessel walls producing plaque. Oftentimes the cardiologist himself is on aspirin, and he even recommends it for his patients with high cholesterol. And if you have a heart attack, then they really assert the benefit of a daily aspirin (or today's latest aspirin substitute drug, the costly blockbuster Plavix®). And if you have artificial valves or cardiac arrhythmia like chronic atrial fibrillation, then the rat poison blood thinner, Coumadin is often prescribed for life.

Aspirin was proven of no benefit decades ago in the *Journal of the American Medical Association* (*Aspirin Myocardial Infarction Study Research Group*). But the Juul-Moller study (*Juul-Moller*) rekindled the practice of prescribing aspirin, even though the research in this study was very faulty. For starters, they did not use aspirin, but Bufferin that contains magnesium oxide, and they also had folks on beta-carotene to simultaneously study cancer prevention. The researchers unscientifically ignored the benefits derived from magnesium (*Pierce*) and that beta-carotene was an antioxidant that could decrease cholesterol deposition (*Riemersma*). **Aspirin users actually had double the normal number of strokes,** as they should when you chemically down-regulate a natural inflammatory reaction meant to protect vessels. Many other errors were detailed in the study and its data analysis elsewhere (*TW*). In addition, 8 studies show aspirin more than doubles the risk of stroke (*He, TW=Total Wellness*).

Aspirin use is the hallmark of a horse and buggy level of knowledge, because Harvard, Tufts University and many other prestigious centers have shown clearly that **vitamin C and vitamin E retard the progression of arteriosclerosis,** which begins with vascular inflammation. They do so by a

36

variety of mechanisms which I don't think you want to hear about (but which include increasing vasodilating nitric oxide synthesis and decreasing intercellular and vascular adhesion molecules) that make cholesterol stick to vessel walls like Velcro. The bottom line is that God's vitamins do a much better job than aspirin, the statin drugs, Plavix and other commonly prescribed synthetic overpriced petroleum-derived chemicals, each having a long list of side effects.

For example, in one study 400 units of vitamin E and 500 mg of vitamin C taken twice daily were compared with the standard treatment in folks who had had heart transplant surgery within the last two years (*Fang*). All patients had a statin drug as well as three immune system-suppressing drugs, corticosteroid, cyclosporine and azathioprine (the latter two are chemotherapy agents, capable of causing cancer, but necessary in transplant patients). Those patients who had the vitamins had decreased thickness of the artery and decreased plaque buildup, compared with those who just had the standard medical treatment with no vitamins.

And these studies are not alone. Many other studies have shown that the two **vitamins, C and E, inhibit plaque growth.** And just giving these two simple vitamins, C and E, made a difference of whether or not you died in ICU (intensive care unit of the hospital) after an accident. **Two inexpensive vitamins, C and E, cut the chance of ICU death 57%!** Yet it's still not routine, in fact, rare is the hospital that even has these vitamins in its pharmacy.

C & E Against Mr. ED

Multiple studies in the most prestigious journals have shown that you can slow down the progress of arteriosclerosis, slow down clotting of vessels, in other words slow down aging and disease progression with mere vitamins C and E. And these studies didn't even look at all the other crucial nutrients that work in harmony in the body. But to turn the poor patient loose by merely recommending he "Take some vitamin E", as many people have told me their cardiologists did, is just as bad as not recommending it at all. For cheap grocery store supplements that list "vitamin E" in their ingredients mean that this is synthetic d,l-alpha-tocopherol. Unfortunately, synthetic vitamin E actually works against any natural vitamin E you might get from your diet or quality supplements. In other words it becomes a negative. Furthermore, real vitamin E is not one thing. It is 4 tocopherols and 4 tocotrienols, so be sure your product has these 8 parts and is not just synthetic, damaging "vitamin E".

Human studies have shown that vitamin E in doses of 400-1000 units a day has not only improved Mr. Ed and high blood pressure, but oxidation of cholesterol that makes it stick to vessel walls like Velcro (*Palumbo, Skyrme-Jones, Barbagallo*). For vitamin E has many mechanisms. It can turn on nitric oxide, as well as being a wonderful antioxidant in the cell membrane inhibiting lipid peroxidation or burning up and premature aging of cell membranes. And it increases levels of the body's detoxifier, glutathione, lowers insulin levels, improves insulin sensitivity, helps the cell maintain magnesium, and more (*Newaz, Barbagallo*). Major problems with many vitamin E studies are they use synthetic vitamin E (d,l-alpha-tocopherol) or only use vitamin E as alpha-tocopherol. Rarely do they add other nutrients. But re-member that although vitamin E has a major role in the cell membrane, it takes 3-6 months to restore the vitamin E. Obviously vitamin E works better when part of an orchestrated symphony of nutrients, the way the body and foods were designed to harmonize, and with all its eight natural parts.

Therefore my personal choice is one **E-Gems Elite** (Carlson, containing the natural tocopherols and tocotrienols) and a quarter teaspoon **Pure Ascorbic Acid Powder** each twice a day. Unfortunately it is my guess that it will be another decade before nutrients are properly looked at. In fact there is an effort to get nutrients off the market. You can understand how this would boost the use of drugs. I'll keep you posted with more heart-saving information in *TW* (*Total Wellness*). Right now drug-oriented practitioners are concentrating on studying or recommending solo rudimentary nutrients, and without the benefit of measuring them in the patient. They just don't appreciate and understand God's beautifully orchestrated plan where the healthful effects of **the symphony of nutrients** are greater than the sum of the parts.   But there's no reason why you couldn't be ahead of the pack and take advantage of this life-saving information.

Many of the nutrients that you learn about here also have the extra-added benefit of decreasing hypercoagulability and decreasing the chance of making blood clots by multiple mechanisms.   Therefore making the recommendation of a daily aspirin shows that these practitioners have failed to keep abreast of the molecular biochemistry literature, and rely on pharmaceutical company-directed practice guidelines, which attempt to make the practice of medicine a no-brainer and require minimal learning time. If you have a cardiologist whom you really like, get him out of the horse and buggy era and onboard the Starship Enterprise. He is so busy learning how to properly code for Medicare and insurance forms that there is little time to learn medicine anymore. Reading this book and *TW* (*Total Wellness*, my inexpensive, referenced subscription monthly newsletter) will save him lots of time and research as it helps him save many lives, the most important one being yours.

Tufts Medical School researchers have shown another nonprescription nutrient helps boost relaxation and expansion of vessels as well as making blood less likely to abnormally clot. And it increases NO (nitric oxide). In yet other ways, this special form of vitamin B3 (niacin) boosts detoxification and the good HDL cholesterol. With its multiple collective mechanisms, it decreases not only high blood pressure, but arteriosclerosis of vessels, claudication (painful legs on walking or climbing), boosts oxygen to the tissues (cutting the need for amputations from gangrene), improves restless legs syndrome, migraines, helps Raynaud's (so does magnesium help this painful fingertips with exposure to minimal cold), and lots more (*Welsh, Sunderland, O'Hara, Kuvin*). For 500 mg of inositol hexaniacinate (non-flush type) niacin, you may want to add **Niacinol** 1-2 a day.

Kill Mr. ED with your DC: the Detox Cocktail

One of the major things that lowers NO, vasodilating nitric oxide, is a heavy dose of naked electrons called free radicals. How do we get them? Through our air, food and water we are continually bombarded by unwanted chemicals that generate disease-producing, age-accelerating free radicals. Our drinking water, outdoor and indoor air, and foods are laden with over 60,000 chemicals, the average person being exposed easily to well over 500 every day. In fact we are the first generation of man ever exposed to such a high level of chemicals in the history of the world. In order to gobble up and neutralize these disease-producing free radicals so they do not further burn holes in and damage the blood vessel endothelial lining causing hypertension, you need a high dose of anti-oxidants that boosts both phases of detoxification, phase I and phase II.

The **Detox Cocktail** is unsurpassed in doing this. This single most important nutrient combination has numerous benefits that we have outlined in *Detoxify or Die*. One of them that I didn't even mention is that the vitamin C component also lowers abnormal blood pressure (*Gokce, Levine, Taddei, Solzbach, Ceriello*), as does another component of the detox cocktail, glutathione (*Meister, Vita, Vaziri*). In addition, the vitamin C in the detox cocktail boosts the glutathione (*Johnston*), by recycling it. And as an extra-added attraction, lipoic acid recycles both of these components, vitamin C and glutathione. So your Detox Cocktail, as well as

√   protecting you from the genetic changes of cancer,
√   lowering cholesterol,
√   revving up your detoxification,
√   boosting longevity, and
√   improving cancer outcomes as just a few of the things your Detox Cocktail does, also does more by
√   lowering blood pressure and
√   protecting your blood vessels from aging and becoming hypertensive.

√ And add to all that its role in protecting every organ from premature degeneration. You really can't afford to be without your daily detox cocktail.

Your **Detox Cocktail consists of 3 ingredients.** Vitamin C is crucial because we don't make it in the body, and cannot eat as much as we need in this world of unprecedented chemical contamination of our air, food and water. As well, it makes the body produce more vasodilating nitric oxide (*Taddei*). The second ingredient, glutathione is made in the body, but it is also lost in the stool or urine with every molecule of chemical we detoxify. I frequently hear folks say they thought that glutathione was not absorbed well orally, but that is not true. In fact, the 800 mg in the detox cocktail is just the right dose to increase plasma levels 2-5-fold (*Hagen*). Frankly, we run out of it much too easily, and when we do, one of the symptoms it creates is hypertension (*Vaziri*). Plus if you are on one of the blood pressure drugs, that lowers your glutathione more, thereby increasing free radicals, which then also raise your pressure, accelerate aging and usher other diseases on board (*Chen*). Lipoic acid is not only a great sponge for sopping up dangerous disease-producing free radicals; it recycles both of these nutrients, vitamin C and glutathione, thus extending their power.

How do you make your own personal Detox Cocktail? It begins with one teaspoon of Ultrafine **Pure Ascorbic Acid Powder.** If it gives diarrhea, cut it back to half a teaspoon. Add the best source of glutathione I know of, **Recancostat,** 400-800mg and **Lipoic Acid,** 300-600 mg. Take this with 1-2 glasses of water since this makes it even more powerful, because water is necessary for all detoxification.

So you have done a great job of boosting your endothelial lining with **L-Arginine Powder, E-Gems Elite,** and your **Detox Cocktail.** Let's see what else you could use if this is not enough. As you will learn, there is a lot that can go wrong with the body to create high blood pressure. The good news is that by finding and fixing as many abnormalities as possible, you help boost the longevity of every single organ of your body, and stop the vicious cycle.

Two Rare Nutrients That Reverse Aging

Mirror, mirror, on the wall, who's getting older and who can forestall? An exciting amount of research by top scientists now clearly explains the molecular biochemistry of aging and eventual disease. The neat part is that we can now translate this knowledge into two simple daily additions/modifications to your Detox Cocktail. First let's focus on the age-defying nutrient, **acetyl-L-carnitine or ALC** for short. This simple amino acid, made in the body out of the amino acids lysine and methionine, is absolutely crucial for carrying fatty acids into the cell's mitochondria where they are turned into the energy to run the body. But most important, it can reverse aging!

One of God's many miracles that scientists have yet to completely fathom is how our food is actually turned into ATP, the biochemical currency of energy that runs the body. Like many other detox nutrients, carnitine gets lower with age and disease. Unrecognized carnitine deficiency can trigger every symptom you can think of whether it's in the weakened weekend warrior trying to get that sport's edge over his playmates to the sickest person on death's doorstep. Carnitine deficiency contributes to every medical problem

43

from hypertension, declining I.Q. and loss of memory to strokes, heart attacks, lung diseases, brain fog, brain loss from alcoholism, chronic fatigue, cancers, to a long list of neurologic diseases from Alzheimer's or mysterious nerve damage like Parkinson's. Every medical problem can be shown to have a deficiency of ALC as a potential component.

One of the first things scientists discovered was that when they restored ALC (acetyl l-carnitine) levels to normal in experimental old rats, it was like turning back the clock. They moved better, their memories were better, they learned new things better, and their heart and blood vessel chemistries returned to more youthful levels. One measurement of aging is damage to the genes inside mitochondria. And we can measure the damage to our genetics. One way is with the 8-OHdG test, which is in your ION Panel. When this is elevated above normal, it means you have sustained increased damage to the genetics in your blood vessels, brain, heart, and liver and may even be headed toward cancer.

But the great news is you can within a few weeks bring this damaged genetic chemistry back to normal with only two non-prescription nutrients, **R-lipoic Acid** and **Acetyl L-Carnitine**. Not only is each nutrient useful in reversing hypertension in those who are deficient (*Houston*), but together they have brought the chemistry and performance of aging rats back to more youthful levels (*Liu, Suh*). Even more interesting was the fact that these two nutrients could stop a lot of serious problems before they occurred. These included, for example, permanent **hearing loss** from prescription drugs like antibiotics, or **heart damage** common after coming off a heart lung machine for bypass surgery, genetic damage from environmental chemicals, or **reversing memory loss** and even preventing fatal heart damage from chemotherapeutic drugs. As well these two nutrients prevent many diabetic complications like cataracts, neuropathy and premature aging via arteriosclerosis as well as high blood pressure. It's foolish to ignore them.

Let's focus on the repair of mitochondria, tiny organelles or kidney bean-shaped packages inside of cells where energy is made. We know two nutrients made in the body can be supplemented, and have proven absolutely key to slowing down aging and even reversing it. Once the mitochondrial genetics are damaged by free radicals, this leads to diseases like chronic fatigue syndrome, excess weight that will not budge, or loss of energy and memory (all usually blamed on aging). Or by interfering with proper fatty acid metabolism, the result can be hypertension. In addition, free radicals in the bloodstream from chemicals in air, food and water burn holes in mitochondrial membranes, damaging the electrical current that runs across this membrane, paralyzing a multitude of chemistries, including the ability of the body to make sufficient energy from fats. These oxidized fats get dumped into our toxic waste storage, the blood vessel lining, creating arteriosclerosis. Two nutrients reverse this.

ALC works in harmony or synergistically with one of the other ingredients that are already in your Detox Cocktail, **lipoic acid**. This universal antioxidant sops up more types of free radicals than any other antioxidant known to man. If this were not enough, it also recycles priceless antioxidants like vitamins C and E plus the detoxifier glutathione, thereby prolonging their useful lives. This nutrient is also crucial in prevention, for example, of nerve damage that leads to impotency, painful peripheral neuropathies and blindness from diabetes. Because it is so potent in protecting from the damage of sugar, it is crucial to incorporate it into a diabetic's regimen, as numerous studies attest. And it not only protects the brain from damage from a variety of neurotoxic chemicals, even poisonous mushrooms (*Amanita*), but reverses the damage done by years of free radicals, called "aging".

Do you think I would teach you about mitochondria if there weren't a very important reason? Leading scientists now know that the **mitochondria are a major site where aging begins,** for this is where energy is created in the body. Unfortunately these little kidney bean-shaped bodies inside of our cells are easily poisoned by ubiquitous plastics and other chemicals that are dumped daily into our bodies (*Melnick*), as described in *Detoxify or Die.* More on that later.

Hottest New Form of Lipoic Acid Now Available

Along with aging comes loss of energy, memory, heart and blood vessel deterioration, and high blood pressure. As you have learned, lipoic acid not only uniquely restores mitochondrial function to youthful levels, but also has actually **reversed the changes of aging** in the laboratory in the test tube. And *in vivo* (in real animals) it has tripled their energy and general metabolic activity, returning the chemistry of rats to more youthful levels. In fact one of the researchers jokingly said the rats were so much more youthful who received R-lipoic acid and acetyl l-carnitine that they were practically doing the Macarena. The exciting part to me is that *the actual form of lipoic acid that was used in these studies to*

46

rejuvenate body chemistry and energy to more youthful levels is now available on the non-prescription market.

Have You Met Rejuvenating R-lipoic Acid?

The regular commercially available form of alpha lipoic acid is a 50/50 racemic mixture of the R and S enantiomers, or mirror images of the lipoic acid molecule. The label merely reads "lipoic acid". The S-lipoic acid form is really a leftover by-product from synthetic production, whereas R-lipoic acid is the pure form found in nature and made in the human body. The R-form is also the one studies that reversed aging were done on and is responsible for most of alpha-lipoic acid's beneficial effects. In fact, R-lipoic acid is the only naturally occurring and 100% biologically active form of al-pha-lipoic acid and *is ten times stronger than the R-S racemate alpha-lipoic acid at reducing inflammation.* All key body en-zymes are structured to hold only the R-form of lipoic acid. Furthermore, as is the case with many synthetic nutrients, the S-form actually interferes with the metabolism of the natural R-form, which has many beneficial actions that are unachievable with the standard alpha-lipoic acid or R/S-lipoic acid.

As another example of its unique potency, R-lipoic acid has actually reversed oxidative stress in aging heart muscles and liver cells. This resulted in *rejuvenated mitochondrial function* that more resembled that of much **younger heart and liver cells.** Furthermore, R-lipoic acid has **reversed mitochon-drial degeneration in brains, bringing them back to younger levels.** And when given orally to rats it has *de-creased lipid peroxidation in brain tissue by 50%.* Translation?

47

It *reverses the changes of aging* in the brain and in the heart and liver! How can we possibly be without it?

R-lipoic acid clearly plays an important role in reversing or at least slowing down the processes we haphazardly call disease and aging. For now, my recommendations would be to take **R-Lipoic 50 mg,** 2 twice a day, once with your detox cocktail and several hours later 1-2 more with your other nutrients. And add one 500 mg ALC (**Acetyl L-Carnitine**) to each dose for reversing or at least dramatically slowing down the aging and deterioration of not only your blood vessels, but heart, brain, liver, eyes, and all other organs (*Suh, Hagen, Lykkesfeldt, Liu*).

Note: A special substitute for R-lipoic acid is the body's first metabolic conversion step, dihydrolipoic acid, DHLA. In fact it is a much stronger antioxidant than commercial synthetic regular lipoic acid (which contains the R and S forms) and the stand-alone R-lipoic acid. This form is especially important for repair of genetic DNA strand breaks (*Suzuki*).
DHLA (Premier Research Labs, Round Rock TX) is safer for allergic folks and since it is nanonized from living sources, has no toxic tag-along, does not eventually damage the cell genetics and other chemistry, as nutrients made in the laboratory can. Use 1/4-1/2 tsp in your Detox Cocktail.

CRP: More Important Than Your Cholesterol

A quarter of a million people die suddenly of a heart attack in the United States each year. But half of them have no common risk factors that would have made anyone suspect they were targets for sudden cardiac arrest. In fact, the truth is that half the people who have sudden heart death never

even had high cholesterol. Researchers know that high cholesterol is "not significantly associated" with sudden cardiac death, but having **high blood pressure doubles your risk of sudden heart death.** Smoking, oddly enough, was not strongly associated with sudden heart attack either, whereas having **diabetes tripled the chance of sudden death.** So doctors studied folks who had sudden cardiac arrests to find out what indicators they did have so that they could identify the people at risk sooner, and help them avoid a fatal heart attack. Another crystal ball test, an elevated **hsCRP** (high sensitivity CRP or C-reactive protein, a marker of inflammation) was the most predictive risk factor (*Albert*). In fact it was much more predictive than the cholesterol level, which is what is commonly used.

It's ironic that at any cocktail party people usually know their cholesterol levels. They erroneously think that this is an important indicator of their heart and vascular health. But a Harvard study shows that it's much more important to know your CRP level, even though most folks sadly have never even heard of it, much less had it assayed. This is also in your **Cardiovascular Risk Panel** (along with the RBC magnesium and your homocysteine level), so you are beginning to appreciate how vital this package of tests is to your longevity and health.

How to Safely Lower Your CRP

You have just learned that a simple and expensive test, called the **hs-CRP or high sensitivity C-reactive protein,** can show that dangerous vascular disease is silently brewing in vessels, even without causing high blood pressure yet. As well it's a crystal ball predictor that diabetes may surface as an elevated CRP nearly triples the risk of developing diabetes, which then in turn accelerates developing heart and blood vessel disease. The recommendations from the *New England Journal of Medicine*, the American Heart Association and other prestigious leaders of how we practice cardiology have suggested that all cardiologists should be measuring this test. Of course, they are still decades behind because along with the CRP should be fibrinogen, vitamin E, testosterone, lipoprotein (a), coenzyme Q10, lipid peroxides, homocysteine, RBC magnesium, testosterone, insulin, and other parameters found uniquely in the **Cardiovascular Profile** (MetaMetrix). For the CRP is only one small piece of the puzzle.

Unfortunately medicine is once more decades late with the necessary information to empower you for a longer and healthier life, and appears to have no intention of telling you how to safely and naturally lower the CRP once you have found it elevated. For it quickly becomes a deficiency of some drug like the statin cholesterol-lowering drugs (Mevacor, Lipitor, Pravochol, Lescol, Zocor), which also have some antioxidant properties. But don't you dare fall for that tale. For they work by poisoning your enzyme in the liver that makes cholesterol. The problem is that you make Coenzyme Q10 with this enzyme (HMG-CoA reductase) as well. And as you will learn later, you need CoQ10 for lots of things, not the least of which is preventing depression, fatigue, gum disease and tooth loss, heart failure, and high blood pressure! Besides, we know all too well how to lower the CRP.

Since the CRP is a major indicator of vascular health, and an elevated CRP indicates inflammation, you want to find the source of that inflammation (*Winslow*). Infection and toxic chemicals lead the pack. Many types of bugs like H. pylori that can silently live in the stomach, cause ulcers, gastritis, or stomach cancer can trigger this inflammation. Or it can migrate to the blood vessels where it causes high cholesterol and arteriosclerosis. An Elevated CRP from infection can be from silent *Herpes simplex* or Chlamydia living in our blood vessels from exposure decades ago. Another common source of bugs that silently infect the heart and blood vessels are the very bacteria in our mouths, in the crevices between gums and teeth or in root canals (*Chase*).

Or an elevated CRP can come from the many chemicals we ingest and inhale like PCBs, dioxins, plasticizers and more that daily stockpile inside our arteries from the air, food and water. For example, if you want to get 500 rats with high cholesterol for drug studies, all you have to do is give them one dose of PCBs (*Mochizuki*). Well, government studies, as I revealed in *Detoxify or Die*, show that 100% of US humans already harbor PCBs, and it happens to be one of the most potent cancer-causing chemicals known to man as well as being arteriosclerosis-propagating.

For toxic chemicals create inflammation via creating naked electrons called free radicals that then drill holes in the coronary arteries and other blood vessels throughout the body. Nature's Band-Aid comes along to plug up the holes so we don't bleed to death. This Band-Aid is cholesterol. You can readily understand that by attacking all high cholesterol with drugs that poison our ability to make cholesterol is like killing the messenger (or more aptly, the Band-Aid). We have failed to deal with the true cause.

Once any inflammation starts, whether it's from a bug or chemical, deficiencies of nutrients fan the fires of inflammation as holes are drilled into the coronary and other artery linings and the cholesterol Band-Aid is called to plug them. Taking the cholesterol-lowering statin drugs is a very dangerous move, for it turns off the enzyme the body uses to make cholesterol. We must have cholesterol for the sex hormones testosterone and estrogen, for the stress hormones like adrenaline, for bile acids so we can absorb our fat soluble vitamins A, D, E, K, plus lipoic acid, beta-carotene, and the essential fatty acids like EPA and DHA, plus coenzyme Q10. Once again you see how **the sick get sicker quicker once they start on the drug merry-go-round.**

Cholesterol-lowering statin drugs put folks on a fast-track for developing an avalanche of degenerative problems including heart disease, cancers, Alzheimer's and much more. They clearly accelerate aging. Plus by turning off the HMG COA reductase enzyme with the statin drug, they turn off your own natural production of coenzyme Q10 which now leads to depression, memory loss, tooth loss, heart disease and much more. Such a bargain! Clever advertising has successfully convinced physicians and patients that high cholesterol is a deficiency of statin drugs. Not true! *Total Wellness 2002-2004* gives directions for non-prescription, safe, no side effects treatments for high cholesterol, which is beyond the realm of this book.

Tocopherol to the Rescue

Even if someone does not have high cholesterol, it is common practice now to put them on the statin (cholesterol-lowering) drug as an antioxidant. But a better choice would be a complete (all eight parts) natural vitamin E like E Gems Elite plus your Detox Cocktail for starters.

For example, vitamin E slows down arteriosclerosis, calcifications, and unwanted clots, plus it down regulates (decreases) the oxidation of LDL cholesterol that transforms it into the form that can attach to blood vessel linings like Velcro (*Devaraj*). And natural source vitamin E, alpha-tocopherol, not only lowers the bad LDL cholesterol, it also turns down the damage from other inflammatory indicators, especially the tumor necrosis factor (TNF) and the CRP (*Devaraj*). But it only happens with vitamin E in the natural form of alpha-tocopherol, not the ineffective synthetic "vitamin E" (d,l-tocopheryl) in cheap grocery store nutrients.

And by the way when you see studies that make the headlines about vitamin E being bad for you, these are usually done with the inferior synthetic vitamin E that is prominent in cheap grocery store varieties. Those studies are right. The wrong kind of synthetic vitamin E is bad for you. But the natural vitamin E (don't forget real vitamin E is 8 things, not just one) has an arm's length of benefits and definitely reverses diseases and promotes longevity.

There is so much unbelievably empowering information that all cardiologists should be telling their patients about. For example, in one study of 900 mg of vitamin E a day, it nearly completely suppressed the uptake into the white blood cells of the bad cholesterol that normally deposits on the coronary lining. In fact vitamin E has done such a great job in preventing the progression of plaque in coronary arteries that it has even done so with patients dumb enough to continue smoking!

In another study, 1200 units of vitamin E a day cut lipid peroxidation, a measure of aging or deterioration of cells from
unavoidable free radicals, by 40%. Alpha-tocopherol (called
vitamin E) is the principal and most potent fat-soluble antioxidant and is mainly located in cell membranes as well as
in the LDL ("bad") and HDL ("good") cholesterol molecules.
White blood cells are the richest source of cytokines (infec-
tion- and cancer-killing substances our cells make to protect
us, resulting in inflammation). Cytokines include substances
like tumor necrosis factor (TNF) and (recall the crystal ball
test) hs-CRP. When the blood carries too much LDL cholesterol, it becomes attacked and oxidized by these cytokines
that are really trying to protect us, hence another reason for
an elevated CRP. And once the cholesterol is oxidized by
free radicals, it glues itself onto the blood vessel lining like a
patch, resulting in arteriosclerotic plaque. As these dangerous electrons eat holes in the lining of endothelial cells,
called lipid peroxidation, this damage pushes Mr. ED (endothelial dysfunction or plain deterioration or rotting of
your silver lining) into more arteriosclerosis and high blood
pressure. But Vitamin E protects against all of this.

Since vitamin E improves vascular disease, it should not
come as a surprise that folks who have high blood pressure
have lower levels of vitamin E (*Wen*). Alone, vitamin E is
not remarkably effective for hypertension, but is necessary
as part of an integrated nutritional program for overall vascular health (*Houston*). Unfortunately most folks are low in
vitamin E because they do not eat whole grains, but instead
the diet is mainly broken grains or flour products. You can
get your vitamin E measured as part of the **ION Panel** that I
will tell you about later. My preferred form of vitamin E?
No contest. The one I recommend, because it uniquely has

all eight components, the four tocopherols as well as four tocotrienols, is Carlson' s **E-Gems Elite**, two a day.

An Odorless Garlic Solution

Some solutions for hypertension (depending on the person) are incredibly easy. For example, how would you like one natural, safe item that not only lowers blood pressure by activating nitric oxide synthase), but has no side effects? And I can throw in a few more benefits. It lowers cholesterol, stops blood from abnormally clotting, lowers homocysteine, revs up an immune system cytokine Il-6, increases blood flow, is a vasodilator and an anti-oxidant, sopping up disease-producing free radicals (*Anim-Nyame*). **Kyolic®** is a proprietary aged garlic, odorless, and proven to do all this and more. I'll tell you more about it in Chapter V. In the meantime, you could use two capsules 2 or 3 times a day or a large squirt of the liquid form instead.

Putting It All Together

I will give you lots of nutritional recommendations in this book, but chances are you don't need them all. You have lots to choose from. Clearly, nutrient deficiencies are epidemic (and so coincidentally is disease). For example, in one study, 61% of the folks who entered the hospital for surgery were deficient in nutrients. And they did not by any means measure the sophisticated ION Panel, meaning they did not actually identify any specific deficiencies. They merely determined they were clinically significantly malnourished. The interesting thing is that being in the hospital was unhealthy for them, because although 61% were malnourished before hospitalization, when they left 82% were! (*Sungur-*

tekin). No wonder 8% died and never made it out of the hospital.

So to treat your endothelial silver lining right and get rid of Mr. ED, you need bare minimum arginine, C, E, GSH, and lipoic acid. You can accomplish that with your nightly Detox Cocktail (GSH or glutathione in the form of **Recancostat, Vitamin C Powder** and **R-Lipoic Acid**) plus all 8 forms of natural vitamin E in the form of **E-Gems Elite** plus L-**Arginine Powder**. You might as well balance it off with a multiple like **Super 2 Daily** or **Heartbeat Elite**. If you want to add extra anti-aging capacity, add **Acetyl L-Carnitine**. Not too difficult for healing the most important organ in your body, that in turn feeds and nourishes every other organ in the body, and for the rest of your life.

Product Sources:

- Ultrafine Pure Ascorbic Acid Powder, Klaire Labs, 1-888-488-2488
- Recancostat, Tyler/Integrative Therapeutics, NEEDS, 1-800-634-1380
- Niacinol, Integrative Therapeutics, NEEDS, 1-800-634-1380
- Lipoic Acid (Metabolic Maintenance) Pain & Stress Center, 1-800-669-CALM
- L-Arginine Powder or capsules, Carlson, 1-800-323-4141
- E-Gems Elite, Carlson, 1-800-234-5656
- Pure Ascorbic Acid Powder, Carlson, 1-800-323-4141
- R-Lipoic, intensivenutrition.com, 1-800-333-7414
- DHLA, prlabs.com, 1-800-370-3447
- Acetyl L-Carnitine, jarrow.com, 1-800-726-0886
- Perfusia-SR, Thorne, 1-800-228-1966, NEEDS, 1-800-634-1380
- Kyolic, Wakunaga, 1-800-421-2998
- ADMA test, metametrix.com, 1-800-221-4640
- Cardiovascular Risk Test, Meta Metrix, 1-800-221-4640
- 8-OHdG (part of ION Panel), MetaMetrix, 1-800-221-4640

References:

Cooke JP, *The Cardiovascular Cure*, broadwaybooks.com, 2003

Valkonen VK, Paiva H, Laaksonen R, et al, Risk of acute coronary events and serum concentration of asymmetrical dimethyl arginine, *Lancet*, 358; 9299: 2127-30, Dec. 22, 2001

Zoccali C, Boger SM, Boger RH, et al, Plasma concentration of asymmetrical dimethyl arginine and mortality in patients with end-stage renal disease: a prospective study, *Lancet* 358; 9299, 2113-24, Dec. 22, 2001

Rector TS, Bank AJ, Spencer H, Randomized, a double-blind, placebo-controlled study of supplemental oral L-arginine in patients with heart failure, *Circulation*, 93; 12: 2135-41, Jun 15, 1996

Gokce N, Keaney JF, Vita JA, et al, Long-term ascorbic acid administration reverses endothelial vasomotor dysfunction in patients with coronary artery disease, *Circul*, 99; 25: 3234-40, June 29 1999

Levine GN, Frei B, Vita JA, Ascorbic acid reverses endothelial vasomotor dysfunction in patients with coronary artery disease, *Circulation*, 96: 11 07-13, 1996

Solzbach U, Hornig B, Just H, et al, Vitamin C improves endothelial dysfunction in coronary arteries in hypertensive patients, *Circulation*, 96: 1513-19, 1997

Ceriello A, Giugliano D, Lefebvre P, et al, Anti-oxidants show an anti-hypertensive effect in diabetic and hypertensive subjects, *Clin Sci*, 81: 739-42, 1991

Vita JA, Frei B, Keaney JF, et al, L-2-Oxothiazolidine-4-carboxylic acid reverses endothelial dysfunction in patients with coronary artery disease, *J Clin Invest* , 101:1408-14, 1998

Johnston CS, Meyer C, Srilakshmi JC, Vitamin C elevates red blood cell glutathione in healthy adults, *Am J Clin Nutr*, 58: 103-105, 1993

Taddei S, Virdis A, Salvetti A, et al, Vitamin C improved endothelial-dependent vasodilatation by restoring nitric oxide activity in essential hypertension, *Circulation*, 97; 22: 2222-29, Jun 9, 1998

Meister A, Glutathione-ascorbic acid antioxidant system in animals, *J Biolog Chem*, 269: 9397-9400, 1994

Duffy SJ, Gocke N, Holbrook M, et al, Treatment of hypertension with ascorbic acid, *Lancet* 354; 9195:2048-9, Dec. 11, 1999

Kumar KV, Das UN, Are free radicals involved in the pathology of human essential hypertension? *Free Rad Res Comm*, 19; 1:59-66, 1993

Newaz MA, Nawal NN, Effect of gamma tocotrienols on blood pressure, lipid peroxidation and total antioxidant status in spontaneously hypertensive rats, *Clin Exper Hyperten*, 21; 8:1297-1313, 1999

Prasad A, Andrews NP, Padder FA, et al., Glutathione reverses endothelial dysfunction and improves nitric oxide bioavailability, *J Am Cardiol*, 34: 507-14, 1999

Kugiyama K, et al, Intracoronary infusion of reduced glutathione improved endothelial vasomotor response to acetylcholine in human coronary circulation, *Circulation*, 97: 2299-2301, 1998

Usala, et al, Decreased glutathione levels in acute myocardial infarction, *Jpn Heart J*, 37: 1 77-1 82, 1996

Wen Y, Killalea, Freely J, et al, Lipid peroxidation and antioxidant vitamins C and E in hypertensive patients, *IJMS*, 165: 210-12, 1996

Houston M, The role of vascular biology, nutrition and nutraceuticals in the prevention and treatment of hypertension, *J Am Nutraceut Assoc*, supplement 1:5-71, Apr. 2002

Das I, et al, Potent activation of nitric oxide synthase by garlic: a basis for its therapeutic applications, *Curr Med Res Opin*, 13: 257-63, 1995

Evans RW, Fernstrom JD, Kuller LH, et al, Biochemical responses of healthy subjects during dietary supplementation with L-arginine, *J Nutr Biochem*, 15: 534-39, 2004

Albert CM., Ma J, Ridker PM, et al, Prospective study of C-reactive protein, homocysteine, and plasma lipid levels as predictors of sudden cardiac death, *Circulation*, 105; 22:2595-99, June 4, 2002

Ting HH, Timimi FK, Creager MA, et al, Vitamin C improves endothelium-dependent vasodilation in patients with non-insulin-dependent diabetes mellitus, *J Clin Invest*, 97:22-28, 1996

Gokce N, Keaney JF, Frei B, et al, Long-term ascorbic acid administration reverses endothelial vasomotor dysfunction in patients with coronary artery disease, *Circul.* 99:3234-40, 1999

Carr AC, Zhu BZ, Frei B, Potential antiatherogenic mechanisms of ascorbate (vitamin C) and alpha–tocopherol (vitamin E), *Circ Res*, 87:349-354, 2000

Fang JC, Kinlay S, Beltrame J, et al, Effect of vitamins C and E on progression of translplant-associated arteriosclerosis: a randomised trial, *Lancet* 359:1108-1113, 2002

Liu L, Meydani M, Mayer J, Combined and vitamin C and E supplementation retards early progression of arteriosclerosis in the heart transplant patients, *Nutr Rev*, 16; 12: 368-3 71, Nov. 2002

Hodis HM, et al., Serial coronary angiographic evidence that antioxidant vitamin intake reduces progression of coronary artery atherosclerosis, *J Amer Med Assoc*, 273: 1849-54, 1995

Salonen RM, Nyyssonen K, Poulsen HE, Six-year effect of combined vitamin C and E supplementation on arteriosclerotic progression: the Antioxidant Supplementation in Atherosclerosis Prevention (ASAP) Study, *Circulation* 107:947-53, 2003

Das I, et al, Potent activation of nitric oxide synthase by garlic: a basis for its therapeutic applications, *Curr Med Res Opin*, 13: 257-63, 1995

Hagen TM. Wierzbecka T, Jones DP, et al, Bioavailability of dietary glutathione: effect on plasma concentration, *Am J Physiol* 59: 524-29, 1990

Shan ZQ, Aw TY, Jones DP, Glutathione-dependent protection against oxidative injury, *Pharmacol Ther* 47; 1:61-71, 1990

Beutler E, Gelbart T, Plasma glutathione in health and in patients with malignant disease, *J Lab Clin Med* 105; 5:581-84, 1985

Ketterer B, Coles B, Meyer DJ, The role of glutathione in detoxification, *Environ Health Persp* 49: 59-69,1983

Plotnick GD, Corretti MC, Vogel RA, Effect of antioxidant vitamins on the transient impairment of endothelium-dependent brachial artery vasoactivity following a single high-fat meal, *J Am Med Assoc* 278:20:1682-86, Nov. 26, 1997

Devaraj S, Jialal I, Alpha tocopherol supplementation decreases C-reactive protein and monocyte interleukin-6 levels in normal volunteers and type II diabetic patients, *Free Rad Biol Med* 29:790-92, 2000

Devaraj S, Harris A, Jialal I, Modulation of monocyte-macrophage function with alpha-tocopherol: implications for arteriosclerosis, *Nutr Rev*, 60; 1:8-14, Jan. 2002

Gregus , Fekete T, Varga F, et al, Dependence of glycine conjugation on availability of glycine: role of the glycine cleavage system, *Xenobiotica*, 23: 141-53, 1993

Temellini A, Mogavero S, Guilianotti P, et al. Conjugation of benzoic acid with glycine in human liver and kidney: a study on the interindividual variability, *Xenobiotica* 23: 1400 27-33, 1993

Chaudhari A, Dutta S, Alterations in tissue glutathione and angiotensin converting enzyme due to inhalation of diesel engine exhaust, *J Toxicol Environ Health*, 9: 327-37, 1982

Fahy O, Tsicopouulos A, Wallaert B, et al., Effects of the diesel organic extracts on chemokine production by the peripheral blood mononuclear cells, *J Allergy Clin Immunol*, 103:1115-24, 1999

Neln A, Diaz-Sanchez D, Saxon A, Enhancement of allergic inflammation by the interaction between diesel exhaust particles and the immune system, *J Allergy Clin Immunol*, 102: 5 39-54, 1998

Peterson G, Saxon A, Global increases in allergic respiratory disease: the possible role of diesel exhaust articles, *Ann Allergy Asthma Immunol*, 77: 263-70, 1996

Perera FP, Molecular epidemiology: insights into cancer susceptibility, risk assessment and prevention, *J Nat Cancer Inst* 88; 8: 496-509, April 17 1996

Ackerson A, Dietary regulation of detoxication, *Altern Comple Ther*, 310-15, Sept/Oct 1996

Manson MM, Ball HWL, Neal GE, et al., Mechanism of action of dietary chemo-protective agents in rat liver: induction of phase I and II drug metabolizing enzymes and aflatoxin B1 metabolism, *Carcinogenesis* 18; 9: 1729-1738, 1997

Heuser C, Vojdani A, Enhancement of natural killer cell activity and T and B cell function by buffered vitamin C (ultra potent-C), in patients exposed to toxic chemicals: the role of protein kinase-C, *Immunopharmacol Immunotoxicol* 19:291, 1997

Lenton KJ, Therriault H, Wagner JR, et al, Glutathione and ascorbate are negatively correlated with oxidative DNA damage in human lymphocytes, *Carcinogenesis* 20; 4: 607-613, 1999

Bates CJ, Walmsley CM, Prentice A, Finch S, Does vitamin C reduce blood pressure? Results of a large study of people aged 65 or older, *J Hypertens* 16:925-32, 1998

Winslow R, Study confirms better predictor of heart risk, *Wall Street Journal*, B-1, Nov. 14, 2002

Chase M, Bacteria behind gum disease are linked to heart-attack risk, *Wall Street Journal*, B6, September 30, 2002

Taddei S, et al, Vitamin C improved endothelial-dependent vasodilatation by restoring nitric oxide activity in essential hypertension, *Circulation*, 97: 2222-29, 1998

Ness SD., Chee D, Elliott P, Vitamin C and blood pressure: an overview, *J Hum Hypert*, 11: 343-50, 1997

Shecter M, Oral magnesium in coronary artery disease: Fresh insight on thrombus in addition, *The Magnesium Report*, 1-4, 1999

Wolf A, Zalpour C, Cooke JP, et al, Dietary L-arginine supplementation normalizes platelet aggregation in hypercholesterolemic humans, *J Am Coll Cardiol*, 29: 479-85, 1997

Chauhan A, More R, Schofield P, Ageing-associated endothelial dysfunction in humans is reversed by L-arginine, *J Am Coll Cardiol*, 28: 1796-1804, 1996

Adams M, Jessup W, Celemajer D, L-arginine reduces human monocyte adhesion to vascular endothelium and endothelial expression of cell adhesion molecules, *Circulation* 95: 662-68, 1997

Bode-Boger SM, Muke J, Frolich JC, et al, Oral L-arginine improves endothelial function in healthy individuals older than 70 years, *Vasc Med*, 8: 77-81, 2003

Gokce N, Keaney JF Jr., Frei B, et al, Long-term ascorbic acid administration reverses endothelial vasomotor dysfunction in patients with coronary artery disease, *Circul*, 99: 3234-40, 1999

Suh JH, Shigeno ET, Morrow JD, Hagen TM, et al, Oxidative stress in the aging rat heart is reversed by dietary supplementation with (R)-(alpha)-lipoic acid, *FASEB J*, 15; 3: 700-706, Mar 2001

Hagen TM, Vinarshy V, Wehr CM, Ames BN, (R)-a-lipoic acid reverses age-associated increase in susceptibility of hepatocytes to ter-butylhydroperoxide both *in vitro* and *in vivo*, *Antiox Redox Signaling*, 2:473-83, 2000

Lykkesfeldt J, and Hagen TM, Vinarsky V, Ames BN, Age-associated decline in ascorbic acid concentration, recycling, and biosynthesis in rats hepatocytes – reversal with (R)-alpha-lipoic acid supplementation, *FASEB J*, 12; 12:1183-89, Sep 1998

Liu J, Killilea DW, Ames BN, Age-associated mitochondrial oxidative decay: Improvement of carnitine acetylate transferase substrate-binding affinity and activity in brain by feeding old rats acetyl-L-carnitine and /or R-a-lipoic acid, *Proc Natl Acad Sci* 99; 4:1876-81, Feb 2002

Hagen TM, Ingersoll T, Lykkesfeldt J, Ames BN, et al, (R)-a-Lipoic acid-supplemented old rats have improved mitochondrial function, decreased oxidative damage, and increased metabolic rate, *FASEB J*, 13:411-18, 1999

Liu J, Atamna H, Kuratsune, Ames BN, Delaying brain mitochondrial aging with mitochondrial antioxidant and metabolites, *Ann NY Acad Sci* 953:133-166, 2002

Liu J, Head E, Ames BN, et al, Memory loss in old rats associated with brain mitochondrial decay and RNA/DNA oxidation: Partial reversal by feeding acetyl-L-carnitine and/or R-a-lipoic acid, *Proc Natl Acad Sci USA* 99; 4: 2356-2361, Feb 19, 2002

Melnick RL, Schiller CM, Mitochondrial toxicity of phthalate esters, *Environ Health Perspect* 45:51-56, 1982

Newaz MA, Nawal NNA, Effect of alpha-tocopherol on lipid peroxidation and total antioxidant status in spontaneously hypertensive rats, *Am J Hypert*, 11: 1480-85, 1998

Newaz MA, Nawal NNA, Gapor A, et al., Alpha-tocopherol increased nitric oxide synthase activity in blood vessels of spontaneously hypertensive rats, *Am J Hypert*, 12: 839-44, 1999

Palumbo G, Avanzini F, Roncaglioni C, et al, Effects of vitamin E on clinic and ambulatory blood pressure in treated hypertensive patients, *Am J Hypert* 13: 564-67, 2000

Barbagallo M, Dominguez LJ, Paolisso G, Effects of vitamin E and glutathione glucose metabolism. The role of magnesium, *Hypertension* 34: 1002-06,1999

Syrme-Jones RA, O'Brien RC, Meredith IT, et al, Vitamin E supplementation improves endothelial function in type 1 diabetes: a randomized, placebo-controlled study, *J Am Coll Cardiol*, 36: 94-102, 2000

Roubenoff R, et al, Malnutrition among hospitalized patients: Problem of physician awareness, *Arch Intern Med* 147:1462-65, 1987

Aspirin Myocardial Infarction Study Research Group, A randomized trial of aspirin in persons recovered from myocardial infarction, *J Amer Med Assoc*, 243:661-9, 1980

Juul-Moller, et al, Double-blind trial of aspirin on primary prevention of myocardial infarction in patients with stable angina pectoris, *Lancet* 340:1421-5, 1992

Pierce JB, *Heart Healthy Magnesium*, Avery Publ, Garden City Park, NY, 1994

Riemersma RA, et al, Risk of angina pectoris and plasma concentrations of vitamins A, C, and E and carotene, *Lancet* 337:1-5, 1991.

He J, Whelton PK, Vu B, Klag MJ, Aspirin and risk of hemorrhagic stroke; A meta-analysis of randomized controlled trials, *J Amer Med Assoc* 280; 22:1930-35, 1998

Hagen TM, Wierzbicka T, Jones DP, et al, Bioavailability of dietary glutathione: effect on plasma concetration, *Am J Physiol*, 259;Gastrointest. Liver Physiol. 22:G524-29, 1990

Kuvin JT, et al, A novel mechanism for the beneficial vascular effects of high-density lipoprotein cholesterol: enhanced vasorelaxation and increased endothelial nitric oxide synthase expression, *Am Heart J*, 144; 1:165-72, Jul 2002

Welsh AL, et al, Inositol hexanicotinate for improved nicotinic acid therapy, *Int Record Med*, 174:9-15, 1961

Sunderland GT, et al, A double blind randomized placebo controlled trial of Hexopal in primary Raynaud's disease, *Clin Rheumatol* 7:46-9, 1988

O'Hara J, et al, The therapeutic efficacy of inositol nicotinate (Hexapol) in intermittent claudication: a controlled trial, *Br J Clin Prac* 42:377-83, 1979

Sungurtkin H, Sungurtekin U, Erdem, et al, The influence of nutritional status on complications after major intraabdominal surgery, *J Am Coll Nutr*, 2; 3:227-32, 2004

Anim-Nyame N, Sooranna SR, Steer PJ, et al, Garlic supplementation increases peripheral blood flow: a role for interleukin-6?, *J Nutr Biochem*, 15:30-36, 2004

Vaziri ND, Wang XQ, Oveisi F, Rad B, Induction of oxidative stress by glutathione depletion causes severe hypertension in normal rats, *Hypertension*, 36:142-46, 2000

Chen N, Liu Y, Greiner CD, Holtzman JL, Physiological concentrations of homocysteine inhibit the human plasma GSH peroxidase that reduces organic hydroperoxides, *J Lab Clin Med*, 136; 1:58-65, 2000

Suzuki YJ, Tsuchuya M, Packer L, Thioctic acid and dihydrolipoic acid are novel antioxidants which interact with reactive oxygen species, *Free Rad Res Comms*, 15:255-63, 1991

Chapter III

An Oil Change for Your Silver Lining

If magnesium correction doesn't stop the spasm of your blood vessels, if adding arginine, vitamin E and the detox cocktail don't do the trick, why are they not enough? Most folks also need an oil change.

The Trans Fatty Acid Travesty

For decades Harvard researchers have been warning the medical profession that a serious mistake has been made by food manufacturers. Real vegetable oils are made from pressing the oil out of seeds like corn, safflower, soybeans, olives, walnuts, coconuts, cottonseeds, flaxseeds and others. But a big problem is that the oil eventually goes bad, and gets rancid and inedible. So chemists discovered in the 1940s that if they heat the oils to over 360 degrees Fahrenheit and added hydrogen molecules, the resulting **hydrogenated oils** would not go bad. But they didn't ask themselves why didn't they go bad. The answer? Because no self-respecting bug would bother trying to eat a "dead" oil. There's little nutrition in it. But that didn't bother the food manufacturers, because they were just tickled to have an oil that would last indefinitely on the shelf and not even need refrigeration. Hence decades ago Mazola oil ushered in the health-damaging era of polyunsaturated hydrogenated oils. And even though Harvard and other researchers warned against them, that they caused high cholesterol and coronary heart disease (*Willett, Longnecker, Enig*), the FDA and medical profession bought it lock, stock and barrel.

Meanwhile not all scientists and physicians were duped into believing that polyunsaturated, hydrogenated Mazola corn oil and eventually most unsaturated vegetable oils should be recommended as healthful. The *Journal of the National Cancer Institute* and also *Cancer Research*, two very prominent cancer journals, contained articles 15 years ago showing that polyunsaturated hydrogenated oils (the ones you commonly buy in the grocery store) act like fertilizer for cancer and make it spread or metastasize. And Harvard researchers showed that these man-made damaged fat molecules of hydrogenated and partially hydrogenated oils act very abnormally when they get inside the human body. They make a beeline for cell membranes but do not act like natural God-given oils. Instead they turn on the chemistry that not only triggers high blood pressure, but arteriosclerosis, epidemic high cholesterol, cancer, diabetes, rosacea, and a multitude of other degenerative diseases (*Chamras*). But the food industry was happy and so was the drug industry. Sales were up. So it was hard to get the attention of the FDA. In fact, even though hydrogenated polyunsaturated oils are clearly known to damage the endothelium, grocery store oils have the FDA's blessing to boast on the package that they contain "healthful" polyunsaturated oils (*Toborek*).

For decades Harvard researchers and other prominent public health groups have warned about the dangers of trans fatty acids that have now literally permeated our food supply. Not only do they lower the good cholesterol HDL by 20% in one study, but also cause constriction as much as 29% in blood vessels. If that were not enough, they raise the levels of the bad cholesterol LDL. And more importantly trans fatty acids are a major cause of the current high cholesterol epidemic (*deRoos*). In fact eating trans fatty acids that have been sneaked into the most seemingly harmless foods, like salad dressings, cereals, breads, French fries, and "healthful" snacks is more damaging than eating saturated fats (*Oomen*). You might as well have a delicious juicy steak than a salad with trans fatty acids in the dressing.

The sad thing is that these oils are hidden in most all salad dressings, chips, dips, pretzels, crackers, cookies, candies, pastries, breads, margarines, cereals, French fries, breakfast tarts, mayonnaises and the majority of processed foods. Packaged foods, snack foods, most all junk foods, pastries and goodies, TV dinners, a vast array of prepared foods, school lunch programs, and restaurant foods contain a large amount of trans fatty acids. They are disguised as hydrogenated and partially hydrogenated vegetable oils, soybean oil, shortening, soy oil, and most other processed oils. If you want to figure out how much trans fatty acid is in a food, look at the label on the back for the calculation of total fats. Then take all the other fats that are listed, add them all together (do not include the total fats) and subtract this total from the total fats. The number remaining is the amount of trans fatty acids hidden in that packaged food.

Even the FDA, which has been notoriously compromised by powerful and expensive pharmaceutical and food industry lobbyists for decades, is now owning up to its obligation decades later to at least make a pretense at protecting the public from trans fatty acids (*Enig, Haley, Angell*). The bad news is the new law for labeling trans fatty acids on foods doesn't go into effect until 2006! Also the FDA regulations allow a manufacturer to blatantly lie to the consumer. He can have 0.5 mg of trans fatty acids per cup serving and write on the label "NO TRANS FATTY ACIDS". This is in spite of the fact that Harvard researchers have shown for decades that *there is no safe level of trans fatty acids in our foods* (*Ascherio*). The FDA condones food manufacturers to lie to us and continue to contribute to disease.

For starters, let's look at some trans fatty acid levels. In one study, trans fatty acids made up as much as 32% of many common foods, with French fries, margarines, crackers and croutons being the highest, 37-41% (*Innis*). In another study, one glazed doughnut gives you six grams (6000 mg!), while a serving of Nabisco Wheat Thins crackers (16 crackers) gives 3.5 grams (3,500 mg!), as does Kellogg's Cracklin' Oat Brand cereal (obviously not a healthful way to start your day), three chocolate chip cookies, two Eggo waffles, or Cheese-It crackers. Still however the food lobbyists won because *manufacturers can put "lean" or "heart healthy" on labels, even if they contain trans fatty acids that are proven to contribute to high blood pressure, high cholesterol, damage the heart and impair chemistry making it difficult to lose weight.* And hospital dieticians recommend processed foods for folks as standard fare in spite of the fact that many scientists have shown, even the smallest amount of trans fats increases the risk of heart disease and other diseases and that **there's no level at which there is no adverse effect** (*Abboud*). So have we gained anything with this upcoming legislation?

I doubt it, but the PR and millions of dollars of regulatory investigation that got us this far makes legislators look good to someone who knows nothing about the real issues. But knowing that more than 60,000 deaths a year can be avoided if Americans quit smoking (*IBD*), doesn't stop the government from subsidizing tobacco growers. So I guess we shouldn't be surprised, since in addition to condoning trans fatty acids, the FDA has approved Olestra (that flat-out stops your absorption of crucial high blood pressure-preventing and cancer-preventing antioxidants like vitamins A, E, D, K, beta-carotene and CoQ10), not to mention crucial medications. In addition, the "scientific studies" blatantly broke the rules of real science, as I'll explain later. Meanwhile be suspicious of foods that boast being "fat-free" or "guilt free". That usually means Olestra is in them, not to mention hydrogenated trans fatty acids as well, making them a double whammy to guarantee developing disease.

Rejuvenate Your Membrane Sandwich
For Delicious Health

So why am I bothering you with all this chemistry? Because the cell membrane, the "skin" surrounding every cell, is the most important part of the human body's communication center. It's the cell's internet, phone system, and cable TV all rolled into one. All the directions coming in and out of the cell have to pass through this membrane. It houses the hormone receptors, the allergy receptors, and releases the cytokines that fight infection and cancer, and makes the prostaglandins to control pain, and much more. It also contains all of the channels that govern the flow of minerals in and out of the cell. And it sends out the minerals, prostaglandins, and other messengers that control blood pressure.

It's too bad that one of the most important and crucial areas of the cell is also one of the first to take a nosedive and deteriorate once we tank up on enough of the trans fatty acids that permeate processed foods. Clearly membrane deterioration underlies every symptom and every disease, especially high blood pressure. The good part is that you and I can correct the damage of a lifetime by giving our membranes a much needed oil change.

If you look at the cell membrane, it is basically a double-layered fatty envelope. If you zoom in with your high-powered microscope I like to think of it as being like a sandwich. The "bread" is mainly the seriously important omega-3 fatty acids called eicosapentaenoic and docosahexaenoic acids (EPA and DHA), but these are kicked out by the trans fatty acids. The "meat" of this sandwich is phosphatidylcholine, but as we age the "meat" layer shrinks (*Yechiel*). The more damaged this membrane sandwich gets, the more quirks in the communication system, hence the more symptoms like high blood pressure and other diseases.

For example, when the calcium channels are finally damaged enough to no longer work properly, you can get high blood pressure, or angina, or congestive heart disease or an irregular heartbeat. But does medicine examine your fatty acids and repair them? No. It sees these as symptoms needing a lifelong prescription for calcium channel blockers. You remember, calcium channel blockers are the classification of drugs most prescribed by cardiologists that are proven to shrink the brain within 5 years. The beautiful thing is that by restoring the membrane's normal function with **Cod Liver Oil** (the best source of EPA and DHA) and phosphatidylcholine (the best source is **PhosChol**), you can reverse a multitude of diseases, including high blood pressure (*Mori, Toft, Morris, Appel, Gundermann*). And phosphatidylcholine's many mechanisms also include protecting against nitric oxide-induced Mr. ED (*Baraona*).

The oil change is so important that in one study of folks 70-83 years old a tiny dose of about 1/4 tsp of cod liver oil improved their blood pressures an average of 14 points! (*Vericel*). Of course, for some that was not enough to totally normalize a significantly higher pressure to start with, but was still a very important drop. Plus remember these researchers were not smart enough to use a real dose, nor correct any of their other deficiencies, much less measure anything. But this sure points out the importance of an oil change. Here folks who have already lived past when most others are dead, made a dramatic change in blood pressure with such a silly under-dose. More on this later.

And don't be confused by all you read until you see the data behind it. For example, you may read in magazines that you should be using polyunsaturated oils, like sunflower oil, to prevent high cholesterol and arteriosclerosis. Should these be your standard cooking and salad oils? Absolutely not! They clearly damage the blood vessel lining and create Mr. ED (*Toborek*). We have really been hoodwinked by the processed oil industry for decades. I've given much evidence in *Detoxify or Die* of how the food manufacturing industry has destroyed the brains and health of millions of Americans through hydrogenated trans fatty acids. As it turns out polyunsaturated oils actually cause inflammation in the blood vessel lining, while olive oil inhibits it (*Carlucci, Toborek, Massaro, Nicolosi*). You're much better off cooking with extra virgin olive oil and using it on your salads. Although a good bottle of olive oil can cost as much as a bottle of wine, there are many great ones for less. Try to always get extra virgin and unfiltered (look for the sediment in the bottom which contains anti-oxidants). Other healthful oils for fun flavors include (non-hydrogenated) **Macadamia Nut**

Oil, Coconut Oil, Walnut Oil, and **Hemp Seed Oil** (sorry, the hallucinogenic part of the marihuana plant is in the flower, not the seed).

And while you avoid the hydrogenated vegetable oils that abound in the supermarkets and in processed foods, you'll automatically be avoiding such things as corn oil, proven to trigger arteriosclerosis (*Hennig*), not to mention that over 40% of it is now genetically engineered. If you can't get to the health food store for cold-pressed organic non-hydrogenated oils, at least use extra virgin olive oil, proven to be much better in protecting against Mr. ED.

As your pressure gets better, you will need to work with your doctor to slowly wean off the medications by three-week intervals. In other words, only make a small dose change every 3 weeks, enabling your body to readjust to re-moval of the enzyme-poisoning drugs. For example, if you have a pill that is unbreakable and only take it once a day, it could be cycled as 2 days on, one day off for 3 weeks. If your pressure is okay, then take one day on and one day off for 3 more weeks, and last, one day on and 2 days off for 3 weeks. Or you could take it every 36 hours instead of 24 for the first 3 weeks, then stretch it to 48. Be sure to monitor your pressure daily. Normal can be anywhere from 110-140 for the systolic (top number) to 50-90 for the diastolic (bottom number), depending on your size and how you feel. But recall you want to aim for 120/75 or less.

Not only does fish oil lower blood pressure (*Morris, Appel*), but vitamin A does in some folks as well (*Toft*). You can do your oil change while you get both nutrients in the form of Carlson's **Cod Liver Oil** (one tsp a day), one of the lowest in toxic heavy metals that I have seen, as well. In addition, your oil change will require you to restore pure phosphatidyl choline in the cell membrane in the form of one teaspoonful of the most potent form I know of, **Phos Chol Concentrate** (Nutrasal). Whenever you give yourself an oil change, you want to also make it easier for these new fats to get into the cell's energy machinery (the mitochondria, where energy is made). You can do that with **L Carnitine** or an even preferred form which goes into the brain cells more easily and is proven to return brain mitochondria to more youthful levels, **Acetyl L-Carnitine** (*Hagen, Ames, TW*).

As well, remember orphan nutrients like phosphatidyl choline in the superlative form of **PhosChol** (Nutrasal) cannot yet be measured, but are absolutely essential for reversing diseases and aging. That's because it rebuilds mitochondrial and all cell membranes and is progressively shrinking from the diet. Therefore you might as well just go right ahead and take it, because I've never seen an excess of it. And just as some folks will never heal until the gut is addressed (since it houses over half the immune system and half the detoxification system, see *No More Heartburn* for details), phosphatidyl choline is another turning point, which can keep someone stalled from total wellness indefinitely. Likewise with all of these chemistries involving fat-soluble nutrients, don't forget your **Bile Acid Factors** or **Super Pancreatin** or **D.A. #34** to improve fat or lipid absorption, especially if you burp a lot (often a sign of a troubled gall bladder).

So How Do You Do An Oil Change?

(1) Stop eating any and all trans fatty acids. That means you have to become thoroughly familiar with their sources and

disguised names. Avoid anything with these words on the label: hydrogenated oil, partially hydrogenated oil, soy oil, soybean oil, vegetable oil, safflower oil, shortening, and cottonseed oil. Only use non-virgin olive oil, **Hemp Seed Oil, Macadamia Nut Oil,** or **Coconut Oil** for cooking provided they are organic, non-hydrogenated cold-pressed oils (see *Detoxify or Die* for more explicit details if need).

(2) Start one teaspoon of **Cod Liver Oil** daily (Carlson brand has sent me their independent laboratory analysis proving undetectable levels of mercury, an important factor). Also use one teaspoon or 3 capsules of **PhosChol** daily, the most potent form of phosphatidylcholine I have found, along with **500 mg** of **L-Carnitine**.

(3) More important would be to have your doctor order the test that looks at your exact level of fatty acids so that the corrections can be tailored precisely to your needs. He merely writes **Fatty Acids** on a prescription blank and you call the number #800 for MetaMetrix for the kit (see Sources at the end of this chapter), and follow the directions. It's very simple, yet health hinges on it.

An oil change takes anywhere from 3-9 months, depending on the severity of your damage and avoidance of trans fatty acids. If you eat out more than once every two weeks, it's very difficult to avoid trans fatty acids without a thorough knowledge of their hidden sources.

Watch Out for Olestra and Other Fake Oils

You've seen the ads and colorful bags at the grocer's. WOW Fat-Free Potato Chips, Doritos, Ruffles, Tostitos and Lay's, and others boasting "fat-free". Laced with Olestra, the chemical that stops you from absorbing fat, they also stop you from absorbing your good fats, like flax oil and cod liver oil. At the same time, Olestra stops you from absorbing your fat-soluble vitamins. So levels of vitamins K, A, D, and E needed not only for healing vessels, but for inhibiting abnormal clotting, cancer protection, osteoporosis prevention, and inhibiting heart disease dive even lower.

On top of that is the fact that pure junk foods with trans fatty acids also have very little real nutritional value of their own, and hook folks on the salty or sugary taste so they don't eat more bland tasting nutrient-rich vegetables. It is tragic that junk foods, loaded with brain- and artery-damaging trans fatty acids, often contain potatoes as well. Most folks with arthritis of any sort do not know that 3 out of 4 who hurt for any reason will stop hurting once they get the potatoes and other nightshades out of their diets (see *Pain Free In 6 Weeks* for details). I can't think of a worse food to send to the public. Yet potato chips, crackers, pretzels and the like are the "fare" on planes, accompanying fast food sandwiches (all with hidden nightshades as well as trans fatty acids) and are common snacks to entertain with.

A plethora of studies show that the very vitamins that Olestra-containing products inhibit the absorption of can cut your cancer and heart attack rates in half. It is mind-boggling how the FDA could O.K. Olestra as a food additive and then viciously attack some nutrients, never letting them return to the market, even after they had been vindicated by multiple studies, as in the tryptophan example. In the meantime, eat as little from a bag, box, jar, can or wrapper as possible. Instead, consume the majority of your food as close as possible to the whole form which God provided. For that is where the maximum nutrition and healing power lies.

And when you see "guilt-free", "fat-free" "reduced fat", "low calorie" or some other enticing buzzword on potato chips, crackers, pretzels, and other snacks, you had better look twice to see if they contain the newer designer fats like Olestra. I'll give you delicious healthful substitutes later. Although okayed by the FDA, this P&G product is a fat substitute that inhibits your absorption of many crucial vitamins. On the outset it sounds really clever to be able to eat fattening foods without gaining weight. But the problem is that by inhibiting the absorption of your fat-soluble vitamins Olestra can foster the development of not only high blood pressure, but heart disease, cancers, schizophrenia, depression, Alzheimer's, Parkinson's and many other diseases. And remember your important fat-soluble vitamins like A, C, D, E, K, beta-carotene, coenzyme Q10 and much more need pancreatic enzymes, bile and other digestive factors in order to be absorbed. Many folks have a long-standing overgrowth of yeasts for example, in the gut that inhibit proper pancreatic and gallbladder function (see *No More Heartburn* for details if needed).

So by allowing Olestra on the market especially when there are already pockets of epidemic deficiencies of many of these vitamins scattered throughout the United States, is a gross injustice. For example, there is already a well-documented epidemic of vitamin D deficiency in the United States. One study showed that Olestra clearly decreases the absorption of vitamin D by 19%, yet the FDA passed it (Jones). This is in a nation that already is plagued by billions of dollars annually in osteoporosis, folks with no teeth leading to poor digestion of foods, plus diabetes, multiple sclerosis, and many other vitamin D deficiency problems, that include high blood pressure, as you will learn.

But that's not the end of the story. Its manufacturer, Procter & Gamble, leaving the fox to guard the hen house, did the majority of studies for this fat blocker, Olestra. And they did some of the most blatantly unscientific studies that I've ever seen in 40 years in the field of medicine. You see, in science when you are examining the properties of anything, nutrients, a medicine, or a substance in foods that blocks the absorption of fats, you give one group of experimental animals the substance and treat the other group exactly the same way, but do not give them the test substance. Therefore the only difference between the two groups is the substance that is being studied. But because P&G knew that Olestra inhibits the absorption of fat-soluble vitamins, A, D, E, and K, they gave these vitamins to the rats that ate Olestra. The study was short so they didn't have time to see what nutrient deficiency symptoms the poor rats would get.

Their "scientific" conclusion should not surprise you. "Olestra is not toxic or carcinogenic when fed to mice in up to 10% of the diet for two years" (*Lafranconi*). This is crooked science at its best, but what's even more discouraging to me is the FDA's scientific specialists hired to protect us passed it. Not only do 15% of the people get diarrhea and other irritable bowel symptoms when they use Olestra (*Hellmich*), but it inhibits the very vitamins that you just learned are needed to stop cancer and heart disease, the number one and two killers in the United States. As well, Olestra can inhibit absorption of some medications which folks depend upon for serious symptoms (*Benmoussa*). This is a travesty, but is unfortunately not a rarity in a political/business world where money talks and honesty takes a real backseat.

Putting the Spark Back In Your Plugs

There are lots of other things that not only repair the blood vessel cell membrane, but make it better than it ever was before. You've been fantastic in learning a lot of molecular biochemistry that most physicians don't know. But when you pass the chemical level, you are next on the electrical level of atoms with orbiting electrons. Just like the computer industry relies on Silicon Valley for its functions, you need silicon to boost your body's electricity. The spark plugs of life depend on a host of minerals, one of which is silicon. With age we tend to get ruptured aortic aneurysms leading to sudden death, burst brain arteries leading to strokes, or torn tendons and ligaments leading to surgery.

And even more important, we get sagging, stretched, dry-looking, wrinkled, lifeless skin as we age, due to loss of glycosaminoglycan-protein complexes and silicon in the matrix of skin and blood vessels. The matrix is the "stuff" in between cells. It is one of the highest silicon-requiring areas of the body, and crucial for cell to cell communication. When it is deficient, cells do not talk to one another and grow wildly. We call this uncontrolled wild growth cancer. Likewise the matrix of blood vessels is the place where we make our own heparin sulfate, God's natural anti-coagulant to protect your blood vessel linings so that they do not accumulate cholesterol, calcium, blood clots and plaque. For when they do they stiffen and stop making protective NO (vaso-dilating nitric oxide gas), then you have Mr. ED. This leads to not only high blood pressure, but also inflammation of blood vessels supplying every organ in the body.

Silica is also crucial in the matrix for holding water, thereby adding flexibility, elasticity or pliability to vessel walls and skin. That's why as people's skin age and they lose silicon, they look drier. In fact, that's what all those expensive cosmetic creams and lotions try to do is re-hydrate the skin. Hoping that the lotions will get absorbed and remain in the skin temporarily, they aim to plump up the skin to give it a more youthful appearance. But the basic problem is that you can't hold the water of youth in skin without enough silicon in the tissues and especially in between cells.

You can refresh your knowledge in *Detoxify or Die* about the other properties of silicon. For it is crucial for the electricity and the communication system between cells. Therefore it is mandatory for healing difficult things like non-union fractures, inhibiting cancers, and much more. Silicon is also used in the brain to inhibit the absorption of aluminum, thereby warding off the damage it causes leading to Alzheimer's.

Most important, silicon has a strong action in protecting arteries from buildup of atheromatous plaque. It is like a Teflon coating making it difficult for calcium/cholesterol plaques to grab onto arterial walls. In one study they measured the levels of silicon in the human aorta with varying degrees of plaque. Normal aortas with no cholesterol, calcifications or plaque had the highest levels of silicon. Whereas the more seriously damaged the aortas were with plaque build-up, the lower the silicon levels were, less than a third of what the healthy ones had (*Loeper*).

In another study, rabbits were given a high cholesterol diet producing plaque in the aortas of 77%. But when they were also given silicon, only 23% developed plaque with the atherogenic diet, and the other 77% were all perfectly healthy in spite of this nasty diet (*Carlisle*). In other studies, the incidence of tumors was higher in animals that had lower levels of silicon. It looks as though silicon is involved in just about every disease from arteriosclerosis to arthritis and Alzheimer's. There are two most potent forms of silica that I know of. The best tablet form is **Cogimax**, containing 50 mg of silica-mineral complex per tablet. The recommended amount is one tablet daily with a large glass of water. Remember to drink at least two quarts of water a day to increase the hydration of your extracellular matrix and keep vessels flexible, not stiff, to prevent high blood pressure, vessel rupture and cholesterol build-up.

The best liquid form I know of is **BioSil**, in the form of well-absorbed orthosilicic acid. Use a large entire dropper-full daily in a glass of water. Shouldn't you start today to plump up aging skin and cholesterol-proof your arteries? For we are all seriously lacking in silica and other trace minerals as the soils get not only progressively depleted with repeated growing, but these important trace minerals are also booted out of the soil by acid rain from the exhaust of factories, incinerators, and the transportation industry.

Also important in the matrix (the stuff between cells), especially of blood vessels, are glucosamine sulfate, chondroitin, and MSM. You thought they were just for bones? No, they keep arteries strong to resist rupture as in strokes and aneurysms. Plus they help make them more resistant to cholesterol deposits and they improve the "elasticity". Glucosamine also increases the vascular matrix production of our own natural anticoagulant, heparin sulfate, thereby retarding arteriosclerosis by yet another God-given mechanism (*McCarty*). Likewise, chondroitin helps boost synthesis of microfibril, a component of vessel elastic tissue (*Kielty*). And don't forget loss of elasticity is a major accompaniment of most tissue aging. An easy way to get them all rolled into one is with **Nutra Support Joint** (Carlson), 2 twice a day.

Trace Minerals

A good companion to all this chemistry/electricity is a mixture of trace minerals. You learned in Chapter I how important the macro minerals are, like magnesium, potassium and calcium. As well, you need selenium, boron, copper, zinc, manganese, molybdenum, chromium and more. Carlson's **Liquid Multiple Minerals** (which are in capsules) make a good source along with your extra magnesium. But there are "trace minerals" other than silicon that also have important (some yet to be discovered) roles inside the healthy vessel.

In *TW*, I've shown lots of evidence in the past how trace minerals like lithium build new brain cells, boron is crucial for healing bone and shrinking the swollen pre-malignant prostate labeled BPH (benign prostatic hypertrophy). Cesium has turned off terminal cancer pain in some and reversed the course of the tumors (described in more detail in *Pain Free In 6 Weeks*), and metals like platinum are used for chemotherapy and gold for rheumatoid arthritis. The bottom line is that these unusual trace minerals are part of normal soil and most likely have roles in our body chemistry that we have not yet discovered.

In addition, missed meals, fast foods, sweating, and worry are just a few of the ways trace minerals are even more depleted. And worse, we do not have readily available measurements of the dozens of rarely heard of trace minerals. Because these trace minerals are progressively lacking in the depleted soils and processed foods, I was happy to find Drucker Labs' liquid multiple minerals specifically formulated with fulvic acids. Fulvic acids are derived from the decomposition of plant and animal tissues in soil, but are smaller in size than viruses and humic acids. Their uniqueness is that they make the minerals highly soluble in a wide range of pHs (*Gaffney*). This means **IntraMin** is able to optimally transport these organic minerals into our tissues, whether alkaline or acidic. The dose of organic **IntraMin** is 2-4 tablespoons 2-4 times a day in clean water.

My experience so far is that these trace minerals attenuate or lessen the loss of other minerals during the far infrared sauna that you will learn about. For example, folks don't seem to need as much magnesium (manifested by undeniable muscle cramping) as they did prior to using the unflavored 100% organic **IntraMin,** containing over 70 plant-derived trace minerals naturally rich in fulvic acid (972-881-2344 or www.druckerlabs.com). I'll keep you posted in *TW* as new data emerges.

Virus Killers,
The Next Cutting-Edge for Vascular Protection

Clearly a major cause of high blood pressure and other diseases of blood vessels is silent virus, bacteria and other infections. In fact the elevated hs-CRP measures this nicely. When viruses infect coronary arteries, they destroy our natural heparin-forming matrix (the space between cells) in blood vessel walls, causing blood clots and fatal heart attacks. As well, latent viruses lurking in many organs and other tissues of the body are a major cause of many types of cancers and other diseases that medicine still tells folks have no known cause and no known treatment. By latent I mean that these viruses can enter the body without causing any symptoms for years, while they silently cause their blood vessel damage. Since we all carry a burden of not only many unwanted chemicals, but also many unwanted viruses, getting rid of these viruses is certainly a goal of mine for you and me.

There are many prescription anti-virals on the market but none are 100% effective, and because they usually work on the genetic material of the virus, they have also the potential of being pro-carcinogens years later in the unsuspecting patient. I would be against taking any prescription anti-viral for myself and family, and certainly would not recommend them to my patients or readers. Therefore I'm on an intense search for natural God-given compounds that have strong antiviral activity especially for vasculitis.

When an infant is born, he does not yet have a reserve of antibodies to protect him against the onslaught of bacteria and viruses that he is going to be exposed to. But God has seen to it that his mother's milk is rich in these protective antibodies, as well as other substances that help fight off viruses. **Monolaurin** is one of these anti-viral agents found naturally in breast milk as well as in amniotic fluid and also in some foods like butter and heavy cream, but especially in coconut oil. In studies performed at the United States government's Communicable Diseases Center, CDC, monolaurin has been able to actually dissolve the protective membrane from 14 types of human viruses (*Hierholzer*). These viruses included measles, flu, herpes simplex, chickenpox, Epstein-Barr Virus, cytomegalovirus virus (a big cause of vascular, brain and heart disease), and SARS-type viruses. **Monolaurin actually disintegrates the lipid envelope or membrane of viruses, destroying their main defense.**

Monolaurin's activity against viruses involves its component lauric acid, binding to the lipid-protein envelope of the virus and inactivating it. By binding to the virus' coat it **prevents the virus from uncoating; now it cannot replicate** and disseminate its infection throughout the body. Also by dissolving the viral envelope, monolaurin inhibits the virus from binding to host cells (your body) and grabbing on for dear life in preparation for releasing an onslaught of virus into your innocent cells. Hence, two mechanisms result from the disintegration of the viral envelope: the virus cannot attach to cells, and it cannot reproduce, since both mechanisms depend upon an intact virus envelope.

Monolaurin 300 mg capsules (Ecological Formulas) are often taken as two capsules three times a day at the first sign of infection and continued for a few days or weeks until the virus is completely gone. It certainly would be a beneficial thing to keep in your emergency non-drug box, especially for the cold and flu season, trying to discourage these bugs from setting up permanent residence in our bodies (*Hierholzer, Ismail-Cassim , Sands, Karbara, Boddie*).

The Silver Solution

When the blood vessel lining (endothelium) gets damaged and weakened by trans fatty acids, it becomes more vulnerable to bugs that set up lifelong infections in arteries, triggering arteriosclerosis. In fact did you know that you can actually "catch" a heart attack? Yes, heartburn can lead to a heart attack. You see, a common stomach bug that causes much heartburn is *Helicobacter pylori*, a bacterium that lives in as much as 2 out of every 3 folks' stomachs. It can live there silently and not cause any symptoms, or it can cause heartburn, ulcers, or rot out the stomach lining, leading to atrophic gastritis, a condition that causes vastly accelerated aging, since you no longer have enough stomach acid to absorb your vitamins and minerals. Or H. pylori can cause stomach cancer, which is on the rise, 8-fold higher in the last two decades, but 43-fold higher if you take the common prescription or over-the-counter acid inhibitors.

You would think that would be enough damage for any ubiquitous bug to cause, but H. pylori doesn't stop there. Once in the stomach, it migrates to the blood vessels of the heart, drilling holes in the lining of the coronaries. Nature's rescue or Band-Aid, cholesterol, appears to plug up the holes so we don't bleed to death. But instead of identifying and killing the H. pylori, we (as usual) kill the messenger. We attack the cholesterol like it's the bad guy, rather than getting rid of the root cause. (You can learn more about H. Pylori in *No More Heartburn*.)

Ubiquitous Herpes virus, H. pylori from the stomach, Chlamydia and many other bugs can eventually end up in the blood vessel wall. Here they are very difficult to get rid of and continually damage the normal function of the blood vessel chemistry, which includes making vasodilating nitric oxide that you learned about in Chapter II. This is where the silver solution might be handy.

For thousands of years silver has been known to have antibacterial properties. Before refrigeration, a silver coin was put in the milk pitcher to keep bacteria from turning it bad. And right up to modern times, silver nitrate drops are used in newborn babies' eyes and silver dressings are used for severely burned patients. As you know, there are lots of silver products on the market touting the ability to kill various bacteria, viruses and protozoa. So how do you sort through the maze? Plus, you say, we have spent so much time teaching you about heavy metals and how to get them out of the body, it seems silly to be putting another heavy metal, silver, into the body. And you are absolutely right. Silver is another heavy metal. That's why the way that it is made is so important for not only excellent antibacterial and antiviral activity, but for keeping it from depositing in your organs and causing heavy metal toxicity and that telltale grayish-bluish skin of silver toxicity called argyria.

Colloidal silver is made with the idea in mind to get as many silver ions into solution as possible to kill unwanted bugs in the body. But this form of silver can also deposit in tissues. In fact you have to shake the colloidal silver bottle before you use it to get the ions more evenly distributed in the solution. Another form of silver however, has been made into much smaller particles, the average size is 0.0008 microns or 8 angstroms. With a particle size this small it means that it has a very high particle dispersion coefficient. Translation: the particle size is so small that it covers a huge area inside and outside of cells, but does not deposit in organs because the huge dispersion coefficient makes a very low dose possible. This type of silver solution has even improved folks with HIV and serious dental infections. It has also been shown to boost the fighting power of white blood cells, especially their antioxidant SOD or superoxide dismutase levels.

This form of silver is so potent that die-off reactions can occur, so merely cut back on the dose. Headaches, joint pains, sweats, nausea, flu-like symptoms, brain fog, fatigue, rashes, itching, chills, diarrhea are the typical types of symptoms that can occur from killing off too many bugs at once. You'll know if it is a die-off because it's self-limited within a couple of days, and cutting the dose or doing your detox cocktail and your detox enema will also terminate the symptoms.

Argentyn 23 provides 23 mg of silver ions per liter and I have seen the independent laboratory data on its ability to kill bacteria. Because of its small molecular size, it cannot be toxic to animals or humans, but the manufacturers sell it only to physicians. I suspect your physician will agree that this subnanometer-sized particle silver preparation should be in your non-drug emergency drug box. The dose of Argentyn 23 for tough infections is a 5 one cc dropper full (5 cc equals one teaspoon) three times a day between meals, and held under the tongue 20 minutes.

For example, although it's beyond the focus of this book, if you are fighting off a bad tooth, I have seen remarkable salvage with the use of Argentyn 23 plus your **QRS Pen** (see *DOD*) or the **Lumen** (see Jan 2005 *TW*) and a couple of immune system-boosting nutrients (we reviewed many in *TW* in the last few years). This is healing after everything else including antibiotics has failed. Plus they were able to avoid root canal or extraction. And remember hidden infection in teeth is a common source of bugs that silently damage blood vessels, especially the coronaries and heart valves.

Remember, when colloidal forms of silver say you must shake the bottle before use, that's because the silver is only temporarily suspended in solution and therefore is capable of settling out as a heavy metal in your body organs. Argentyn 23 has no such requirement and therefore fewer side effects. Because it is in a small molecular form, it effectively kills bugs while it avoids depositing in and damaging your cells. Argentyn 23 has proven to fight off some of the nastiest viruses such as HIV and herpes and is being considered as a treatment for the SARS Coronavirus, especially when it mutates. Shouldn't it be part of your non-drug emergency drug box? It is in mine. And more importantly, we need this safer form of silver to get hidden bugs out of our silver linings.

So there you have why and how to do an oil change, simple version or elaborate. Whichever you decide, do it. For as you will learn in the next chapter, the everyday chemicals that we all have in us damage the chemistry and conversion of DHA, the most important fatty acid in the brain, heart, and blood vessel membranes. So even though you take cod liver oil that contains it, it's not a guarantee that it all gets properly metabolized. The resulting unsuspected deficiency of the fatty acid, DHA, is a main initiator of not only vascular disease, but heart diseases of all types, cancer and most degenerative diseases. Plus, as a major control of gene repair, hidden DHA deficiency is a crucial contributing cause of accelerated aging (*Verlengia*).   But we have the tools to identify and totally correct this problem, bringing you to new levels of wellness. So let's continue.

Product Sources:

- Hemp Seed Oil, intensivenutrition.com, 1-800-333-7414
- Macadamia Nut Oil, MacNut Oil, 1-888-350-8446
- Coconut Oil, prlabs.com, 1-800-370-3447
- Coconut Oil, Bio-Tech, 1-800-345-1199
- Cod Liver Oil, carlsonlabs.com, 1-800-323-4141
- PhosChol, nutrasal.com, 1-800-364-4416
- L-Carnitine, jarrow.com, 1-800-726-0886
- Nutra Support Joint, carlsonlabs.com, 1-800-323-4141
- Fatty Acids Blood Test, metametrix.com, 1-800-221-4640
- IntraMin, druckerlabs.com, 1-972-881-2344
- Monolaurin 300 mg, Ecological Formulas, 1-800-275-3495
- Argentyn 23, Natural-Immunogenics, 1-888- 328-8840
- Bile Acid Factors, Jarrow.com, 1-800-726-0886
- Super Pancreatin or D.A. #34, Carlson, 1-800-323-4141
- QRS Pen, High Tech Health, 1-800-794-5355
- Lumen, lumenphoton.com, 1-828-863-4834

References:

Rentz EJ, Viral pathogens and severe acute respiratory syndrome: Oligodynamic Ag+ for direct immune intervention, *J Nutr Environ Med*, 13; 2:109-1 18, June 2003

Hall, RE, Bender G, Marquis RE, Inhibitory and cidal antimicrobial actions of electrically generated silver ions, *J Oral Maxillofacial Surg*, 45: 783, 1987

Russell AD, Path FR, Hugo WB, Antimicrobial activity and action of silver, *Prog Medic Chem*, 35: 352, 1994

Thurman RB, Gerba CP, The molecular mechanisms of copper and silver disinfection of bacteria and viruses, *CRC Crit Rev Environ Control*, 301, 1989

Oka H, et al., Inactivation of enveloped viruses by a silver-thiosulfate complex, *Metal-Based Drugs* 1; 5-6: 511, 1994

Montes LF, Muchinik G, Fox CL, Response to varicella-zoster virus and herpes zoster to silver sulfadiazine, *Cutis* 38; 6: 3635, 1986

Feng Q, Wu , Chen GO, et al, A mechanized study of the antibacterial effect of silver ions on *Escherichia coli* and *Staphylococcus aureus*, *J Biomed Mater Res*, 52: 662-68, 2000

Goetz A, Tracy RL, Harris PS, Oligodynamic effect of silver, *Silver in Industry*, NY, Reinhold 402-3, 1940

Von Nageli C, On the oligodynamic phenomenon in living cells, *Denkschriften der Schweiz Naturforsch Ges*, 33:174-82, 1983

Antelman M, Multivalent silver bacteriosides, *Precious Metals*, 16:151-63, 1992

Antelman M, Anti-pathogenic multivalent silver molecular semiconductors, *Precious Metals*, 16: 141-49, 1992

Antelman M, Silver (II, III) disinfectants. *Soap/Cosmetics/Chemical Specialties*, 52-9, March 1994

Greer N, Silver and its compounds. In: Block S (ed.) *Disinfection, Sterilization and Preservation.* Philadelphia: Lea & Ferbiger, 380, 1983

Shimizu F, Shimizu Y, Kumagai K, Specific inactivation of *Herpes simplex* virum by silver nitrate at low concentrations and biological activities of the inactivated virus, *Antimicrob Agents Chemother*, 10; 1:57-63, 1976

Coleman VR, et al, In vitro activity of silver sulfadiazine aginst herpesvirus hominis, *J Infect Dis* 132; 2:79-81, 1973

Edwards-Jones V, Foster HA, Effects of silver sulphadiazine on the production of exoproteins by *Staphylococcus aureus*, *J Med Microbiol*, 51; 1:50-5, Jan 2002

Elia V, Niccoli M, Thermodynamics of extremely diluted aqueous solutions, *Ann NY Acad Sci*, 827:241-8, June 1999

Fox CL, Silver sulfadiazine, a new topical agent for *Pseudomonas* in burns, *Arch Surg*, 96:184-8, 1968

Jansen B, et al, In vitro evaluation of the antimicrobial efficacy and biocompatibility of a silver-coated central venous catheter, *J Biomater Appl*, 9; 1:55-70, Jul 9994

Berger TJ, et al, Electrically generated silver ions: quantitative effects on bacterial and mammalian cells, *Antimicrob Agents Chemother*, 9; 2:357-8, 1976

Berger TJ, et al, Antifungal properties of electrically generated metallic ions, *Antimicrob Agents Chemother*, 10; 5:856-60, Nov 1976

Wlodkowski TJ, Rosendranz, HS, Antifungal activity of silver sulphadiazine, *Lancet*, 2; 7831:739-40, Sept 1973

Bragg PD, Rainnie DJ, The effect of silver ions on the respiratory chain of *Escherichia coli*, *Can Microbiol*, 20:883-9, 1974

Zhao G, Stevens SE, Multiple parameters for the comprehensive evaluation of the susceptibility of *Escherichia coli* to the silver ions, *BioMetals* 11:28, 1998

Becker R, Spadaro JA, Treatment of orthopedic infections with electrically generated silver ions, *J Bone Joint Surg*, 60:871-81, 1978

Dean W, et al, Reduction of viral load in AIDS patients with intravenous mild silver protein, three case reports, *Clin Prac Altern Med*, spring 2001

Modak SM, et al, Combined use of silver sulfadiazine and antibiotics as a possible solution to bacterial resistance in burn wounds, *J Burn Care* 9; 4:359, July/August 1988

Jansson G, Harms-Ringdahl M, Stimulating effects of mercuric and silver ions on the superoxide anion in human polymorphonuclear leukocytes, *Free Rad Res Commun*, 18; 2:87-98, 1993

Carlucci N.A., et al, Oleic acid inhibits endothelial activation, *Arterioscler Thromb Vascular Biol*, 19:220-28, 1999

Toborek M, Lee YW, Garrido R, et al, Unsaturated fatty acids selectively induced an inflammatory environment in human endothelial cells, *Am J Clin Nutr*, 75: 119-25, 2002

Massaro M, Carlucci MS, DeCaterina R, Direct vascular antiatherogenic effects of the oleic acids: a clue to the cardioprotective effects of the Mediterranean diet, *Cardiologia*, 44:507-13, 1999

Nicolosi RJ, Woolfrey B, Fosher R, et al, Decreased aortic early atherosclerosis and associated risk factors in hypercholesterolemic hamsters fed a high- or mid-oleic acid oil compared to a high-linoleic acid oil, *J Nutr Biochem*, 15: 540-47, 2004

Gaffney JS, Marley NA, Clark SB, eds., *Humic and Fulvic Acids*, ACS Symposium Series #651, American Chemical Society, Washington D.C. 1996

Toft I, Bonaa KH, Jenssen T, Effects of n-3 polyunsaturated fatty acids on glucose homeostasis and blood pressure in essential hypertension, *Ann Intern Med* 123; 12:912-18, Dec 15, 1995

De Roos NM, Bots ML, Katan MB, Replacement of dietary saturated fatty acids by trans fatty acids lowers the serum HDL cholesterol and impairs endothelial function in healthy men and women. *Arterioscler Thromb Vascul Biol*, 21; 7: 1233-37, July 2001.

Oomen CM, Ocke MC, Kromhout D, et al, Association between trans fatty acid intake and 10-year risk of coronary heart disease in the Zutphen Elderly Study: a prospective population-based study, *Lancet* 357: 9258: 746-51, Mar. 10, 2001

Mori TA, Bao DQ, Burke V, Beilin LJ, et al, Docosahexaenoic acid, but not eicosapentaenoic acid, lowers ambulatory blood pressure and heart rate in humans, *Hypertension* 34; 2: 253-60, 1999

Benmoussa K, Sabouraud A, Bourre JM, et al, Effect of fat substitutes, sucrose polyester and tricarballyate triester, on digitoxin absorption in the rat, *J Pharm Pharmacol*, 45; 8692-96, Aug. 1993

Lafranconi WM, Long PH, Wooding WL, et al, Chronic toxicity and carcinogenicity of olestra in Swiss CD-1 mice, *Food & Chem Toxicol*, 32; nine: 7 89-98, Sept. 1994

Jones DY, Miller KW, DeLuca HF, et al, Serum 25-hydroxyvitamin D concentrations of free-living subjects consuming olestra, *Am J Clin Nutr*, 53; 5:1281-87, May 1991

Hellmich N, Consumers sink teeth into olestra chips, *USA Today*, 6 D, Sept. 30, 1996

Loeeper J, Goy-Loeper J, Rozensztajn L, et al, The anti-atheromatous action of silicon, *Atherosclerosis* 33: 397-408, 1979

Schwartz K, A bound form of silicon in glycosaminoglycans and polyuronides, *Proc Nat Acad Sci*, 70: 1608-12, 1973

Carlisle EM, Silicon as an essential element, *Fed Proc*, 33: 1758-1766, 1974

Carlisle EM, Garvey DL, The effect of silicon on formation of the extracellular matrix components by chondrocytes in culture, *Fed Proc*, 41:461, 1982

Carlisle EM, Discussion. In *Silicon Biochemistry* (Ciba Foundation Symposium 121) 228, 1986

Chamras H, Ardashian A, Heber D, Glaspy JA, Fatty acid modulation of MCF-7 human breast cancer cell proliferation, apoptosis and differentiation, *J. Nutr Biochem* 13: 711-716, 200

Anonymous, Trends and innovations, *Investors Business Daily (IBD)*, A2, July 2, 2003

Abboud L, The truth about trans fats: coming to a label near you. FDA orders disclosure of more details on packages; a new excuse to eat Cheetos, *Wall Street Journal*, D1, July 10, 2003

Fairfield KM, Fletcher RH, Levinson W, Vitamins for chronic disease prevention in adults: Scientific review, *J Am Med Assoc* 287; 23: 3116-3126, Jun 19, 2002

Morris MC, Sacks R, Rosner B, Does fish oil lower blood pressure?: A meta-analysis of controlled trials, *Circulation*, 88:523-33, 1993

Appel LJ, Miller ER, Seidler AJ, Whelton PK, Does supplementation of diet with "fish oil?" reduce blood pressure? A meta-analysis of controlled trials, *Arch Intern Med*, 153:1429-38, 1993

Gundermann KJ, ed., *The "Essential" Phospholipids as a Membrane Therapeutic*, Polish Section of European Society of Biochemical Pharmacology, Institute of Pharmacology and Toxicology, Medical Academy, Szczecin, Poland, 1993

Ascherio A, Willett WC, Health effects of trans fatty acids. *Am J Clin Nutr.* 66:1006s-1010s, 1997

Parker-Pope T, Food makers race to drop trans fats, but some substitutes aren't much better, *Wall St J*, 8/10/04, D1

Baraona E, Zeballos GA,Lieber CS, et al, Ethanol consumption increases nitric oxide production in rats, and its peroxynitrite-mediated toxicity is attenuated by polyenylphosphatidylcholine, *Alcohol Clin Exp Res*, 26: 880-89, 2002

Hierholzer JC, Kabara JJ, In vitro effects of monolaurin compounds on enveloped RNA and DNA viruses, *J Food Safety*, 4: 1, 1982

Ismail-Cassim N, et al, Inhibition of the uncoating of bovine enterovirus by short chain fatty acids, *J Gen Virology*, 71: 10: 22 83-9, 1990

Sands J, et al, Extreme sensitivity of enveloped viruses, including *Herpes simplex*, to long-chain unsaturated monoglycerides and alcohols, *Antimicrob Agents Chem* 15; 1:67-73, 1979

Karbara JJ, Lipids as host-resistance factors in human milk, *Nutrit Rev* 38: 65, 1980

Boddie RL, Nickerson SE, Evaluation of postmilking teat germicides containing Lauricidin, saturated fatty acids, and lactic acid, *J Dairy Sci*, 75: 6: 1725-30, 1992

Enig M, *Know Your Fats*, 1-301-680-8600 or bethesdapress.com, 2000

Verical E, et al, The influence of low intake of n-3 fatty acids on platelets in elderly people. *Athersclerosis*, 147:187-92, 1999

McCarty MF, Glucosamine may retard atherogenesis by promoting endothelial production of heparan sulfate proteoglycans, *Med Hypoth*, 48; 3:245-51, Mar 1997

Kielty CM, Whittaker SP, Shuttleworth CA, Fibrillin: evidence that chondroitin sulphate proteoglycans are components of microfibrils and associate with newly synthesized monomers, *FEBS Lett* 386;2-3:169-73, May 1996

Innis SM, Green TJ, Halsey TK, Variability in the trans fatty acid content of foods within a food category: Implications for estimation of dietary trans fatty aid intakes, *J Am Coll Nutr*, 18; 3:255-60, 1999

Willett WC, et al, Intake of trans fatty acids and risk of coronary heart disease among women, *Lancet* 341581-5, 1993

Longnecker MP, Do trans fatty acids in margarine and other foods increase the risk or coronary heart disease?, *Epidemiol* 4:492-5, 1993

Verlengia R, Gorjao R, Curi R, et al, Comparative effects of eicosapentaenoic acid and docosahexaenoic acid of proliferation, cytokine production, and pleiotropic gene expression in Jurkat cells, *J Nutr Biocemh*, 15; 657-65, 2004

Hennig B, Reiterer G, Robertson LW, et al, Dietary fat interacts with PCBs to induce changes in lipid metabolism in mice deficient in low-density lipoprotein receptor, *Environ Health Persp*, 113; 1: 83-87, 2005

Chapter IV

The Heavy Metal Connection

It has been known for decades that the stockpiling of cadmium in the kidneys causes high blood pressure. Where does it come from? It is unavoidably ubiquitous in our foods. You can't get away from it even if you eat organically (although it should reduce it). It comes from industrial and auto exhausts primarily. It spews out of smokestacks and tailpipes, is taken up into clouds then rains out into soil and streams where plants and animals concentrate it before we eat them. And cadmium isn't the only heavy metal in the environment that can tank up in the kidneys and create hypertension. Lead, mercury, arsenic and other heavy metals have the ability to damage kidneys. Yet there is more. They can all damage the endothelial blood vessel lining, damage enzymes crucial in maintaining normal blood pressure, and damage the channels in cell membranes of blood vessel and heart cells so that calcium, magnesium, potassium and other minerals do not flow the way they should, another mechanism to cause high blood pressure! (*Salonen, Guallar, Lustberg, Kopp, Moller, Schwartz, Chai, Cheng*).

For example, just having a blood lead level that is "normal", but at the high end of normal, increases your chance of cancer 68%, increases your chance of early death from any cause by 46% and death from cardiovascular disease 33% (*Lustberg*). It took decades before scientists began to realize that the cut-off for lead was too high for children to have normal brains and intelligence (*Bellinger*). Not only are scientists discovering that "normal" blood ranges of heavy metals are much too high for healthful longevity, but that unsuspected heavy metals are the cause of much cardiovascular disease, especially high blood pressure (*Lin*). It is especially imperative to correctly assay for lead if a patient has hypertension because it can not only destroy the kidneys (*Tsaih*), but also destroy brain function (*DOD, Tsaih, Lin*).

Lead that silently stockpiles in our bodies goes on to contribute not only to high blood pressure, but diabetes and kidney disease necessitating renal dialysis (*Tsaih*). But like many heavy metals, this is not easy to find with just a blood level, because that's not where the majority of it hides. It hides out in the bones. Unfortunately as folks age, they tend to get lower in minerals, leading to bone loss and osteoporosis. Along with this, the heavy metals start to leach out of bone storage and land in important organs, like blood vessels, heart, kidney and more, triggering high blood pressure, heart disease with various names like angina, arrhythmias or congestive heart failure, or they get cancers from these heavy metals, too. So how do we identify then get rid of the heavy metals and restore normal blood pressure?

Rescue for the Stranded Illness

Often folks do all sorts of things that have worked for other folks, but to no avail. They are still not well. Is your blood pressure up regardless of what you do? Do you feel like you have been sentenced to a lifetime of blood pressure pills. Or for that matter do you have any other illness that is at a standstill? Are you unable to get to a higher level of wellness and off the drug merry-go-round? If you are stranded with the label of high blood pressure, or any other medical label that is going nowhere, you most likely have *heavy metal syndrome*. You need **accelerated heavy metal detox**.

There was a time when the only heavy metal I had ever heard about was a rock group. But the sad thing is that we are the unique generation that has the highest levels of hidden heavy metals in the history of man. "What?" you say, "I hardly had any heavy metals when I did the ION Panel". What you need to understand is that this shows the heavy metals that are only in equilibrium inside your red blood cells. The body tries to stuff undetoxified heavy metals away in as many other organs as possible to dilute the effect for any one organ. The biggest repository is bone. The next may be our blood vessels.

Another reason you may have a false sense of low heavy metals from your RBC results is there are no normal people with negative levels anymore. So the test shows where you are relative to others, the population average. Therefore, even if you are on the low side of normal, if you add the results of your cadmium to your lead, to your mercury, to your arsenic, you will see that your total load might be off the page. Your total toxin level of just 4 heavy metals is a pretty serious burden for the body to bear. Just imagine what else lurks in the body that you haven't seen, for you have only peeked at less than a half dozen. In order to see the nasty hidden heavy metals that are just screaming to get out of your whole body, you need to do a **heavy metal provocation test**. Begin by choosing one out of many substances that drag heavy metals out of their hiding spots in your brain, heart, liver, kidneys, bones, etc. and push them out through the urine and stool. When you do this, you invariably find large amounts of all sorts of heavy metals that really cannot be found in any other way. Best of all getting rid of them reverses high blood pressure and a variety of other previously unconquerable diseases.

Quick Silver, Slow Death

Mercury, known as quick silver in former times, is a prime example of a heavy metal and how it sneaks into the body and causes disease. As I showed in *Detoxify or Die*, even babies in the Arctic born to their Eskimo mothers have surprisingly high levels of mercury, PCBs and other brain-damaging chemicals in their bodies. As well, even the mother's breast milk contains them. We have successfully polluted the entire world. For example, the majority of power plants for electricity in the U.S. and throughout the world are coal-fired, and mercury is spewed into the air as a side effect of this. It drifts out miles away in clouds and rains bring it to the soil and streams. From here plants and animals accumulate these chemicals and we eat them, stockpiling them in us as their last toxic stop. Still you may not be impressed with the dangers of mercury toxicity, so let me add, that it does not just come from our country.

Mercury Toxicity is Going to Become Even More Epidemic

If you thought that mercury toxicity has been solved, guess again. Sure, our government is recommending people only eat fish once a month because of dangerous mercury toxicity in our streams, lakes and oceans. But the misinformed ADA (American Dental Association) is still crucifying dentists for removing mercury "silver" amalgam fillings, another major hidden source (see *DOD*). Yet there's an even bigger problem.

The developing countries are learning their lessons well from the U.S. on how to pollute the world. For example, China because of its cheap labor, has become our surrogate, the recipient of many of our factories for production of "American" goods. The problem is she is growing so fast and voluminously now that it has required an enormous boost in the production of electricity. This is provided by burning coal and is adding immensely to the toxic world-wide mercury burden. The mercury spewed forth from these power companies is taken up into the clouds and has been proven by Harvard scientists, for example, to rain out over the United States (*Pottinger*). Collectively we have so polluted our oceans that every country has folks who are polluted with mercury. Even the pristine Arctic folks and polar bears are not exempt from mercury toxicity.

And in China mercury pollution is rising at such fast rates that there are whole towns where folks suffer from mysterious neurological symptoms traced (when they have been among the lucky few to have it investigated) to insidious mercury poisoning. Lenient government regulations have allowed Chinese power plants to pay small fees for the privilege of polluting and not having to use expensive air scrubbers on their smokestacks, saving them millions of dollars. Meanwhile, some grains from nearby fields contain over 40 times as much mercury than grains from less contaminated areas.

In 1989 Dr. William Rea (the foremost clinical ecologist in the world, to whom most doctors send their failures) and Dr. Theron Randolph (the father of chemical sensitivity) and I lectured for three weeks in six cities in Chinese medical schools and hospitals. We saw firsthand how they live. My heart goes out to people living, working and eating in these polluted areas, for most haven't a clue as to why they're so desperately ill with symptoms rendering drugs powerless, or why their young children are suffering brain loss or mysteriously dying of cancers.

This conveyor belt of bad air dumping on the U.S. will inevitably raise the hidden mercury levels even higher, bringing more damage and disease to folks while shortening their lives. In fact U.S. government studies now show that one in six babies born in the United States has brain damage from collective common environmental pollutants. The sad fact is that we have progressively less control over the sources. For example, 80% of our goods are made in China, or at least parts of them, and the China/US trade gap is expected to double (*Eig*). **Over a third of our environmental mercury now comes from other countries, and it is slated to rise dramatically (*Pottinger*).**

With mining, manufacturing, incineration, electricity generation, soil and food contamination plus dental silver/mercury amalgams, there is no way heavy metal toxicity isn't going to exponentially increase as other developing countries follow. Our medical profession should be right on top of it and yet rarely is a single heavy metal measured. Every doctor should know the facts that are in *Detoxify or Die*, yet sadly it is not part of standard medicine to look for any toxicity, much less heavy metals. Those of you like myself who have suffered with and subsequently recovered from mercury toxicity know how it can easily destroy a life. On the flip side, we know what it feels like to be reborn once it has been removed and the damage has been repaired.

This finding, reported in the very first column on the front page of the *Wall Street Journal*, should be a blatant warning to the field of medicine and yet I doubt it will make a significant difference. In January the EPA released research indicating nearly a million babies born in the U.S. between 1999-2000 had unsafe levels of mercury in their blood. The same *Wall Street Journal* article went on to tell about a National Hockey League defenseman who began suffering dizziness, headaches, insomnia and blurred vision forcing him to miss 25 games. Luckily he found a doc smart enough to measure his mercury levels which were abnormally high because of his daily tuna fish.

Meanwhile some grain fields in China contain nearly 40 times the amount of mercury that other fields do. While major drinking water reservoirs in China have 18 times the EPA's recommended levels of mercury, which are considered safe. And you know from following the *TW* newsletters and our other books over the last decade and a half that many "safe" levels are eventually found to be too high and actually unsafe. Plus don't lose sight of the fact that we are talking about one pollutant, one heavy metal, not your total daily dose of invisible disease-triggering pollutants. If you think heavy metal toxicity does not affect you now, just wait, for it will inevitably affect all of us, and the increased vulnerability of infants and children means the intellect of our future generations is in great jeopardy (*TW* 2003-5).

In the meantime, consider us an elite privileged group just to be aware of the scope of this on our future health. Heavy metals in blood vessels and kidneys are an important, yet ignored cause of high blood pressure, regardless of age (*Sorensen*). And it will only get worse. Luckily it is reversible. But without this awareness, all the medical care and drugs in the world are powerless to actually cure your high blood pressure or anything else you might get from your lifetime accumulation of heavy metals. Luckily, we know how to cure ourselves.

Many people like myself developed our initial mercury toxicity from the "silver" amalgam mercury fillings in our teeth. This has been one of the most damaging blunders in the medical/dental world. Not only to put so much mercury in people's mouths, but to ignore the oceans of evidence proving that it could be the underlying root cause of so much medical misery for decades (references in *Detoxify or Die*). And there are multiple other sources for mercury contamination in the body. It is a preservative in immunizations, and old time teething powders contained mercury, as did hemorrhoid creams and skin bleaching creams. Mercury was a common fungicide in paints and it out-gases from home walls where it was used. It's in the ballast of fluorescent lights. And as deadly as it has been for many, it is only one of thousands of toxins that EPA scientists have discovered that we have accumulated in our bodies in this century. For once we take it in, we rarely have enough detoxification capability to get rid of all we stockpile every day.

As bad as mercury is, it is only the tip of the iceberg, for we are a veritable garbage pail of all sorts of heavy metals. We all have lead in us, but most of it is not detectable by blood test. It is stored in bones and other organs like the heart and kidneys where it also can cause high blood pressure as well as numerous other diseases from lowering of IQ to cancers. In fact, lead **raises the homocysteine levels** that then increase your chance of early heart attack, cancer, Alzheimer's, as well as adult blindness from macular degeneration and much more (*Schafer, Homocysteine Collaboration, Rodrigo, Nash*). Lead is a major factor in the progressive elevation of blood pressure as well as deterioration of brain function. And stored lead may be the reason why some people cannot correct their homocysteine levels with nutrients. And when you do have blood levels drawn, research shows that the "normal" level or safe cut off is grossly too high. Low levels can severely damage the brain of infants, children as well as adults (*Canfield*). Let's get the lead out!

Provocation Test Shows Heavy Metal's True Colors

So if common blood levels are useless for assaying heavy metals, how do we find out what is lurking beneath the surface poisoning us? You need to do a provocation test to force the heavy metals out of hiding. To do this test, merely have your doctor write a prescription for two **Nutrient & Toxic Elements 24-hour urine** tests (MetaMetrix). After you have called the 800# to get your kits from MetaMetrix, first collect 24 hours of urine while taking none of your nutrients. You could use either 2 **Captomer** (250 mg each) 3 times a day for three days, or if you prefer and have paid prescriptions, 5 **Chemet** (100 mg each) three times a day. Both require medical supervision. Remember to be off your nutrients when taking a chelating drug, because you don't want to be chelating out the minerals you just took.

On the second day of Captomer or Chemet while you are still taking it, begin your second collection for a 24-hour urine. After the second 24-hour urine has been collected, you do not need to continue the Captomer or Chemet. When you compare the lab results of your before and after taking the detox substance to pull heavy metals out of hiding, you will be amazed at how much your body is eager to get rid of. Even in folks who have been aggressively detoxifying for several years and have made great strides in their health, I've been startled by the remaining heavy metals that come pouring out. Of note is that many heavy metal detox specialists are now satisfied that two 8 hour urine collections are sufficient (versus two 24-hour collections), and that certainly makes it less complicated, not having to lug your urine jug to work.

As huge amounts of heavy metals pour out of hidden areas of the body, one problem is they have to go through the kidneys to get into the urine. But the kidneys in many folks (especially those with high blood pressure) are usually already loaded with cadmium and other heavy metals. In order to minimize the stress on the kidneys, an old Edgar Casey remedy is useful. Get top-quality **Castor Oil** (Premier Research Labs). Put a couple of ounces on six layers of organic cotton (which you can get from Premier Research or use old organic cotton pillowcases) folded to make a pad about 6 by 4 inches. Put this over the kidney area for about an hour. A heating pad can improve the effectiveness. Your kidneys are in the midline on either side of your spine at about waist level. Although I only have anecdotal evidence, and have not done studies or found any supporting scientific evidence, I think it has merit in improving the circulation, blood flow and detoxification of the kidneys when they are overloaded. Also adding one teaspoon of **L-Arginine Powder** to a glass of water three times a day further protects the kidneys from heavy metal overload (*Andoh*).

Once you understand how many heavy metals are still blocking your chemistry, it is then easy decide on a program to continually get them out of your body at a much-accelerated rate. I would not recommend taking the Captomer more than three or four days in a row without giving yourself a break of eleven or more days off before cycling again. If you are highly sensitive, you may need to cut back the dose to as little as a 100 mg Chemet or Captomer one day a month. If you are otherwise vigorously healthy and on the other end of the spectrum, that would allow you to use as much as 500 mg three times a day for four days on, and eleven days off. It's imperative to titrate your tolerance.

Remember to have no nutrients when you're taking the Captomer or Chemet because you want to pull out heavy metals secretly stored in your body. You do not want to waste it on pulling out nutrients that you took that day. It is important to do your detox cocktail once a day (Chapter II, or see *Detoxify or Die* for more details) when you are taking the Chemet or Captomer. On the days that you are off the Chemet or Captomer, then you want to replenish your minerals vigorously as though you had done a sauna (described later here and in more detail in *Detoxify or Die*). For heavy metal detox medicines also pull out good minerals like magnesium, zinc, chromium, calcium, and much more. Clearly, you may do your detox cocktail and detox enema daily, whether you are on or off the medicines.

After several months of this you may want to take a rest from your detox program for a month or more. Then it is a good idea to repeat your 24-hour urine collection while taking Chemet or Captomer and see what else your body is eager to get rid of. You see, it takes a while for the body to readjust and equally disseminate the heavy metals throughout again. For example, you may be surprised that mercury was your highest heavy metal in the past but now it is arsenic or lead. The body has a certain order in which it wants to get rid of its heavy metals and oftentimes you won't know that other damaging heavy metals are present until you have gotten rid of the ones that the body wanted to get out first. You are forced to respect this innate pecking order.

We are so loaded that it literally takes many people years of this program to get to a disease-reversing low level of heavy metals. But just think of the unbelievable advantages of putting your body back to a level of heavy metals where it was 20 or 30 years ago or even better than when you were born, since many babies are born with excessive heavy metals on board. I can't emphasize too much how important it is to get rid of these heavy metals, since they sit right in enzymes and actually boot out the minerals that normally sit in those enzymes to make them work. Having heavy metals sit in enzymes in place of, for example zinc, paralyzes the enzymes so they cannot work properly and instead accelerate aging and the development of all diseases.

There are three reasons why identifying and reducing silently stored heavy metals is so important.
• Many folks will never get better until they do it.
• Many folks will not live long enough to detoxify with diet, nutrient corrections and sauna only. They are just too sick and too polluted.
• And since we are continually tanking up on heavy metals, we need a program that will get rid of heavy metals at a faster rate than we are accumulating them.

This has been one of the major ways to bail folks out of that dark abyss where they have been told "There is no known cause and no known treatment for what you have". Give it some serious thought for yourself. I'm continually astounded at how high the levels are even in "clean, detoxi-fied, asymptomatic people". They are an accident waiting to happen. Whether you are unhealthy or well, it makes sense to do this. And since it can be ultra-titrated to the most sensitive person, this adds another distinct advantage.

Note: If your doctor is reluctant to prescribe heavy metal chelators, have him read this plus *Detoxify or Die* (presti-gepublishing.com or 1-800-846-6687), which has more scientific evidence and explanation. Once he sees the compelling logistics he will want to do it for himself and his family, as well as you.

Diagnostic Provocation Program
And Accelerated Heavy Metal Detox

1. Order 2 test kits for 24-hour urine for Toxic Elements.
2. Read all instructions that accompany the test kits.
3. Before the first urine test is started, discontinue any supplements for 2 days prior. Do not collect the first urine of the day (morning). Start with the second urine of the morning and continue throughout the day for a 24-hour collection (or you may opt for the shorter 8 hour collection).
4. Start whatever detox medication you have been prescribed (Chemet, Captomer, Detoxamin etc.,) for 3 days. Also use the Detox Cocktail (Chapter II) with no other supplements. You may boost the detox cocktail with glycine, taurine, and L-arginine. Do the detox enema daily (see *Wellness Against All Odds* for maximum details).
5. The second urine test is started on day 2 of taking the detox medicine. Do not collect the first urine of the day (morning). Start with the second urine of the morning

and continue throughout the next day for a total of 24 hours (or the optional 8 hours).
6. Call the # 800 for pickup of both urine tests.
7. Schedule with your doctor to go over the results of your tests and how to proceed. Meanwhile you may continue the basic protocol, 3-4 days on and 11-30 days off. When off detox for 11-30 days, take your usual supplements, the detox enema plus your Detox Cocktail:

Bare minimum your daily nutrients should also include:

Detox Cocktail (Chapter II)
- 1/2 to 1 teaspoon of pure Vitamin C Powder
- 50-100 mg R-Lipoic or 300-600 mg Lipoic Acid
- 400-800 mg Recancostat or 500-1000 mg NAC

Plus
- 1-3 teaspoons daily of Cod Liver Oil
- 1-2 capsules daily Carlson Super 2 Daily
- 1 capsule daily B-Complete-100 (Carlson)
- 2 capsules daily E-Gems Elite (Carlson)
- 2 capsules daily Liquid Multiple Minerals (Carlson)
- 1-4 tbsp. IntraMin (Drucker Lab)
- 1 capsule daily Chelated Zinc 30 mg
- 1 capsule daily Chelated Chromium 200 mcg
- 2-4 capsules daily PhosChol 900 (Nutrasal)
- 1 capsule daily Chelated Manganese 20 mg (Carlson)
- 1 capsule daily Selenium 200 mcg (Carlson)
- 1 cc 2 times a day of prescribed Magnesium Chloride Solution or non-Rx Natural Calm, 1 teaspoon twice daily, or another form of magnesium amounting to 400-800 mg a day.

Heavy Metal Detox Program

Are you ready to start a 3-6 month Accelerated Heavy Metal Detox Program? Let's solidify your understanding. For 1-4 days while you are on the chelation drug or suppository use:

Detox Cocktail:
- 1/2-1 teaspoon of pure Vitamin C Powder
- 300-600 mg Lipoic Acid
- 400-800 mg Recancostat or 50-100 mg R-Lipoic Acid
- 8-16 ounces of filtered water

Add detox medications for your Accelerated Heavy Metal Detox Program:
- 1-2 capsules, 2 times a day of **Captomer** 250 mg (or Chemet 100 mg, 2-5 capsules twice a day). Or you may opt for 1-4 **Detoxamin Suppositories**, as you will learn later. **No other supplements should be taken when on detox medications.** However you should stay on prescriptions and discuss with your doctor how detoxification may change your medication levels.
- Daily use your detox enema and detox cocktail.
- If you go too fast or too long, you will feel worse, so back off to the dose where you feel fine. Maybe you can only do one Captomer or Chemet once a day versus the maximum of 2 Captomer 250 mg 2-3 times a day x 4 days. The minimum is 1 Chemet a month, maximum is 5 Chemet 3 times a day x 4 days on and 11 days off. Perhaps you can only take 2 Chemet twice a day for 2 days a month, so be it. Never make yourself worse. Remember if you are on Captomer, it is 2 1/2 times stronger than Chemet so the dose is adjusted down accordingly.

- Then for 11-30 days stop the Captomer, Chemet, Detox-amin, or whatever you use for accelerated heavy metal detox. Continue the detox enema, Detox Cocktail, and now resume your supplements.
- Also during the 11-30 days off the detox medications, you will need to take extra nutrients for 1 week, in addition to your usual supplements, to make up for the extra good minerals that the detox medications deplete:
- Extra minerals to be taken above and beyond your regular nutrients for one week after taking detox medications:
  - 1 capsule Carlson Super 2 Daily
  - 1 capsule Liquid Multiple Mineral (Carlson)
  - 1 capsule Zinc Balance (Jarrow)
  - 1 capsule Chelated Chromium 200 mcg
  - 1 capsule Chelated Manganese 20 mg
  - 1 capsule Selenium 200 mcg (Carlson)
  - 1 capsule Moly B (Carlson)
  - 1 tablet Iodoral (Optimox), needs a prescription
  - 1 capsule Boron, 3-6 mg daily (Pure Encapsulations)
  - 1 cc twice a day of either Rx Magnesium Chloride Solution or 1 teaspoon twice a day of Natural Calm, or other source of 400 mg magnesium a day
  - 2 tablespoons of liquid trace minerals, like IntraMin (druckerlabs.com or 972-881-2344)
  - 4-9 capsules PhosChol daily
  - 1 capsule Vanadyl Factors (Jarrow)

As well, when you are getting rid of minerals, you want to remember to periodically boost minerals that are not readily measured but highly essential. The products I have found useful include not only the liquid trace minerals **IntraMin** (multiple organic trace minerals), but **Iodoral** (a special form of iodide/iodine that boosts failing thyroids), for iodine deficiency is rarely tested but is another hidden epidemic deficiency. Unsuspected iodine deficiency fosters thyroid disease with weight gain, sluggishness, constipation, depression, exhaustion, hair loss, and more.

Note: Iodoral sometimes requires a prescription and can be obtained through Belmar Pharmacy (303-763-5533). If your physician has the slightest hesitation to prescribe it for you, share with him the convincing data and references in the Iodoral article in November 2004 *Total Wellness*.

Boron is needed for not only strong blood vessels, but also bones. Use **Boron** 2-6 mg a day for the boosting weeks. Also silicon is needed for blood vessels, brain function and energy. Use **BioSil** (that you have learned about) or **Cogimax** (neglected trace silica minerals that are especially important in building strong blood vessels). Cogimax does not require a prescription, and is from the same company, Optimox, that makes Iodoral, 1-800-223-1601.

Summary: Heavy Metal Detox Protocol

The basic program for 3-6 months can appear difficult, so let's just summarize it in yet a different way:

You are merely 1-4 days on the Accelerated Heavy Metal Detox Program, using detox medication, Detox Cocktail, and no supplements. The Detox enema must be done daily during this period. This is followed by 11-30 days of the Detox Cocktail plus supplements, but no detox medication. *Detox enema is advised but not mandatory during this period.* So basically you are on the detox medication or your nutrients, but not both, but regard less of which phase you are in, you always do your daily Detox Cocktail and Detox Enema.

So how can you tell if healing is stalled because unseen levels of heavy metals are socked away in crucial organs? The best way to identify them is to have your doctor write a prescription for two 24-hour urines for **Toxic Elements** (Meta-Metrix). When you receive your kits, collect the first 24-hour urine, and merely stay off your nutrients the day before and the day of the collection.

The second collection is a little trickier. You can call NEEDS for **Captomer-250** (Thorne) or get your prescription for Chemet or use non-prescription **Detoxamin suppositories**, which you will learn about later. Take up to two Captomer 100 mg three times a day with two 8 oz. glasses of water (spring water, not mineral water) and if you suspect you are really toxic or chemically sensitive, use the Augmented Detox Cocktail below twice a day (versus the regular detox cocktail). Stop all your nutrients for three days, from the day before to the end of the second urine collection. Instead to the Detox Cocktail with 800 mg of **Recancostat**, 50-100 mg of **R-Lipoic Acid**, one teaspoon of **Ultrafine Vitamin C Powder**, the Augmented Detox Cocktail may also include the addition of one each: 500 mg **Taurine**, 500 mg **Glycine**, 1-2 **Thisilyn**, 2 **IndolPlex**, and 1/2 teaspoon **L-Arginine Powder** (Carlson).

What's the purpose of all this? The first urine shows the amount of heavy metals that you are able to get rid of on a daily basis and the test includes much more than mercury, cadmium, lead, arsenic, and aluminum. If you have ordered **Nutrient and Toxic Elements** as opposed to just **Toxic Ele-**

ments, you will also see how much of the "good" minerals you lose with chelation.

Meanwhile, in comparison to the first urine, the second urine shows what your body is eager to get rid of once you drag the nasty heavy metals out of their hidden organ storage sites and dump them into the urine. Most people are amazed to find that their levels of silently sequestered heavy metals are enormous, usually off the page. This explains why you have not been able to get beyond your current point of stalled healing progress. For many, now is the time to make the life-changing and life-saving decision to go into an accelerated heavy metal detox program, getting rid of the heavy metals a lot faster than you had been.

Now you could do intravenous chelation for four-hour sessions four times a week in some chelation doctor's office, but it is much cheaper and easier to do it orally (or rectally, as I will show you shortly). Once you know that your stumbling block is hidden heavy metals and that you have to get rid of them a lot faster, use the accelerated heavy metal detox protocol with your chelation of choice, titrated to your tolerance, for 1-4 days.

Then follow your 1-4 days of detox with 11-30 days of no chelation, so that now you can restore your nutrient levels. You may also use your augmented detox cocktail and detox enemas whether you are on or off chelation. To your regular nutrients add the extra nutrients as described above for at least a week after every chelation session, to make up for the good minerals that were lost.

What is the point of all this? You want to aggressively rip those hidden heavy metals that are stored in multiple target organs out of their safe storage and dump them into the urine. So use plenty of water and the detox cocktail with L-Arginine Powder so that these heavy metals do not get hung up in the kidneys and damage them any more than they already have (*Andoh*). You will be rebuilding and fortifying your nutrients as usual during the time off chelation. So the cycle is 1-4 days on and 11-30 days off and you keep cycling like this for about 6 months and then recheck your **RBC Minerals** to be sure you have not lost too many minerals, and your **Toxic Elements** to determine what is left to get rid of. You may need to do this for more than 6-12 months before you reduce your levels to where your health takes a quantum leap or new turn, and symptoms begin to melt away.

Caveats

Some important caveats when you do this protocol is to do it with your doctor's supervision and have him check a chemical profile and GTT once every few months to be sure you are doing it properly and not damaging your liver or kidneys. For example, if you just rely on the standard chemical profile's BUN (blood urea nitrogen) to diagnose kidney damage, you'll be sorely disappointed. For studies show that you can damage 75% of the kidneys before the BUN is abnormal. However the GTT is a much more accurate and early indicator of not only liver damage but also kidney damage (*Kramer*).

Because Captomer is the same as the prescription drug Chemet (both are DMSA), if you have paid prescriptions, your doctor can save you money by writing for Chemet. But remember it is very expensive and only comes as 100 mg so you have to increase the level accordingly. If he won't do it, have him read *Detoxify or Die* as well as this. If nothing else he should want to do it on himself and that will be a good teaching tool for him.

Chemet is a prescription drug (used mainly for children with lead poisoning) and Captomer is the same chemical, but 2 1/2 times stronger, and less expensive, unless you have paid prescriptions, of course. It has just as many potential side effects as any other drug with headaches, arrhythmias, gut symptoms or even death. But I sincerely wonder how many of the reported symptoms for children using it were actually symptoms brought on by taking the drug without all the precautions and nutrient replacements of the accelerated detox program described here. For the detox cocktail and detox enema, for example, are rarely done even though they can greatly reduce serious symptoms.

For example, the majority of doctors treating kids for lead poisoning are adhering to the old outdated standard (as I've shown you in *TW*) where they think that the kid is safe if his lead is under a level of 20. Therefore they are treating only highly poisoned kids. But they do so without ever measuring (much less correcting) their detoxification minerals, fatty acids, vitamins, or amino acids. So they have huge amounts of lead pouring out of kids' brains and into their kidneys, hearts and other organs without making sure it goes to the urine and doesn't damage other organs. These kids may be too low in certain detox nutrients to totally get rid of their heavy metals, but these are rarely checked in these studies or in real life detoxification. Also rather than only 1-4 days at a time, many of the docs in the studies treat little kids for two weeks at a time which is ridiculously scary when you're not using any detox nutrients and you're dealing with a youngster with an immature detoxification system. But such is the field of medicine that prefers to remain totally unschooled in proper detoxification biochemistry.

After several months of the detox protocol you will want to check your **RBC Minerals** again also because this oral chelation pulls out good things like zinc, chromium, calcium and magnesium, as well as the health-damaging heavy metals. Also this protocol would be absolutely contraindicated if you were pregnant or nursing or had any known liver or kidney problems (without strict medical supervision). The beauty of it is that it dramatically carries people over the hurdle that was keeping them from getting progressively better. They now can heal the impossible. And many folks frankly have too high a level of toxins to be able to live long enough to get rid of them by any other slower method.

Another place where you might be hoodwinked is if you don't understand the rebound phenomenon. Once you have dramatically reduced your level of heavy metals, you may anxiously check your blood levels. But they may be low now and then in a few months they may be higher than they were before. Or other heavy metals that were low before may now be elevated. The reason? After you have pulled enormous amounts of heavy metals out of their sequestered sites in various organs, the body tries to equilibrate. So when you check the RBC heavy metals you may find that now there are even higher levels, since they have been further pulled out of storage from formerly toxic organs. I personally think this is a protocol that we should do at least a

few times a year for life. Why? Because we are forever being polluted with heavy metals from an ever-increasing array of unavoidable sources.

Also if you find you still have, say too much mercury on
board, you may need to switch to Chemet or Captomer for a
while, since these are made of DMSA, a chemical that is
better at removing mercury than is EDTA, that you will
shortly learn about. Your physician should guide you with
these more precise decisions after you have made a significant dent in your heavy metals and other foreign chemical
loads.

Clearly **heavy metal detoxification has caused a major
quantum leap in health,** unattainable any other way. And it
doesn't matter how sick or how well you are. There have
been folks rescued from the brink of death as well as honed
athletes who have improved their edge on competitors. The
aggressive lowering of huge amounts of hidden heavy metals has turned around the worst heart diseases or improved
memory, mood and IQ of those who are well. If you are not
convinced to do this now, perhaps you should turn around
and read it again, or put it inside your calendar and read it
again in a few months when you are less stressed. It is one
of the most important decisions of your life.

Why Is Taurine So Important?

Taurine is a simple amino acid that basically we do not make
enough of to keep up with our detoxification needs. If that
were not enough reason, it also makes up our bile which is
needed to emulsify and absorb healing fats like Cod Liver
Oil and fat-soluble vitamins A, D, E, and K, plus CoQ10 and

B-carotene. Furthermore, taurine is important for not only turning off high blood pressure in susceptible folks by itself, but for reversing high cholesterol, arrhythmias (irregular heartbeat), congestive heart failure, seizures, eye problems, and much more, since its highest concentrations are in the heart, brain and eye.

Taurine works at lowering blood pressure by many mechanisms. It can detoxify chemicals that cause hypertension, stabilize the cell membrane, augment magnesium's actions, reduce homocysteine, cause vasodilatation, reduce claudication (pain in legs on walking), promote diuresis (fluid loss), and stop platelets from abnormally clumping and causing thrombophlebitis (blood clot in veins), strokes or heart attacks (*Houston, Nakagawa, Kohashi, Trachtman*). And taurine is often low in hypertensives, which you can discover from your amino acid levels in your **ION Panel** and confirm with a therapeutic trial (*Kohashi*). A normal dose is **Taurine 1000 mg,** 1-2 twice a day.

Chelation: Detoxification in Vain?

For decades folks have literally saved their lives with IV chelation. Many of these folks have had blood pressure resistant to any medications, intractable angina or end-stage heart failure and were doomed for an early death. With IV (intravenous or given in the vein by needle) chelation of calcium disodium ethylenediaminetetraacetic acid (CaNa2EDTA) given slowly over three or four hours at a dose of usually two to three grams, folks have literally been given a new lease on life. It works by not only pulling out heavy metals from damaged hearts and heart valves, but it pulls heavy metals out of storage in blood vessels, kidneys, and more, and it has even pulled out calcifications of arteries. Although it has been a miracle for many, like anything else it has its disadvantages:

- You need a chelation physician in your city, and many folks have had to travel several hours to find one.
- Once you get there, chelation is usually 3000 mg and lasts three or four hours and is done two to four times a week for 30-60 or more weeks.
- By forcing a chelation dose of 3 gms on the body over a short period of time, it puts more stress on organs, like the kidneys, and has caused kidney failure.
- The cost is usually over $150 per session, not counting travel and time lost from work.
- Blood studies reveal that plasticizers from the IV bags and tubing accumulate in the bloodstream and later end up contaminating the rest of the human body. These plastics from IVs often end up in the peroxisomes, little organelles inside of all cells (except mature red blood cells because they have lost their nuclei). They quietly damage the chemistry needed by all cell membranes and thereby lead to further diseases, including high blood pressure (references in *DOD*).

So as life saving as EDTA chelation has been, it is time-consuming, difficult, unphysiologic, potentially dangerous and expensive. You might say it is detoxification done in the veins. But due to all these negatives, it is really done (pardon the pun) in vain. Who needs all the disease-producing phthalates and to force the system and risk renal damage?

But fortunately a method of using patented chelation suppositories has opened up the whole world of heavy metal detoxification, making it available to everyone. The very same chemical that goes into the IV, CaNa2EDTA (calcium disodium EDTA) has been incorporated into rectal suppositories in a smaller dose so that it does not put so much strain on the system, especially the kidneys. A suppository contains 750 mg of calcium disodium EDTA (about a quarter of a regular IV dose), which is slowly absorbed through the sigmoid colon during the night and gently works detoxifying the body of its heavy metals. This avoids the disadvantages I've shown you for IV chelation and by using a gentler dose every night, you allow the body catch-up time. Let's look at all of the advantages to this method:

- You save money and time as well as the danger of traveling.
- You lose no time from work or home.
- You are gently coaxing the heavy metals out of the body with a quarter of the dose you would be given with the IV method. This relieves the kidneys and rest of the body from the strain of forcing a higher dose on it over a shorter period of time.
- It is extremely inexpensive, the cost of the suppositories for nightly chelation for a month can be approximately what you would pay for one chelation session. *If you mention this book when you order, they will give you a discounted price.*
- There are no disease-producing plastics or phthalates to be absorbed, since there are no IVs.
- You have total flexibility with the dose. You can use half or a quarter of a suppository or two or three of them at a time. Likewise you can chelate on the days that you want to and forget it on the other days. For example, you could chelate on the even days and correct your mineral deficiencies on the odd days. Or you could chelate for a

week and then be off for a week, boosting your minerals aggressively during that time.

Always during chelation of any sort you still need to periodically take extra minerals as I described earlier, because EDTA chelates out some of your good minerals as well as your heavy metals. The name of the suppository that is so safe and affordable is **Detoxamin**, available from World Health Products, 16285 South 125 East, Salt Lake City, UT 84020, 877-656-4553, web site microzyme@mindspring.com. It will revolutionize medicine.

Note: You could do your heavy metal provocation test with 4 Detoxamin suppositories daily for 2 days; 2 twice a day (like 10 p.m. and 2 a.m.) collecting the 8-hour urine on the second morning, or spread 4 suppositories out through each of the days preceding and during the urine collection. This would be in place of the Captomer or Chemet, with 4 Detoxamin suppositories daily being equivalent to one daily standard IV chelation dose (assuming you have a healthy colon and have absorbed it all). I personally think that the availability of this product will force medicine to acknowledge the importance of dealing with heavy metal toxicities that underlie most diseases. My hat goes off to the **Detoxamin** Company for researching and making chelation available, affordable, non-prescription, and practical for a greater number of people. For as you have learned, heavy metal toxicity is at the root of many incurable conditions, and it is not going to go away.

Not only does CaNa2EDTA have a long history of reversing all sorts of cardiovascular diseases including hypertension, angina, claudication, congestive heart failure, and arrhythmias, but also for dissolving occlusive plaques that were blocking important neck, heart and leg vessels and where surgery was contraindicated (*Riordan, Blumer, Gordon, Cranton, Halstead, ACAM courses, Olszewer, Rudolph, Chappell, Kindness, Gooneratne*). It removes cholesterol plaque and lowers cholesterol (*Uhl, Mariani, Mitchell, Rosenma, Schroeder*). And don't forget that EDTA is the same chemical they put in blood tubes in the laboratory to keep blood from prematurely clotting (*Toyota*). Yet EDTA is so safe that it has been a FDA approved food additive for over 40 years (*Oser, Davidson*).

A couple of other products merit mention. For someone who needs a much lower, more delicate dose for titrating or needs EDTA chelated with magnesium, there is 100 mg magnesium EDTA suppository called **Medicardium** (*Wartman*). Again you can tailor the dose to your needs.

DetoxMax Plus is another promising product, especially for those not wanting a rectal suppository form of chelation. It is oral EDTA that normally is only 5-15% absorbed. But this form is a sonicated micronized form of EDTA coupled to phosphatidylcholine, magnesium and lipoic acid that serve not only to facilitate assimilation, but to remove cholesterol from storage sites in arterial walls (*Yechiel, Bar, Samochowiec, Howard, Stafford*). It has provided remarkable improvement for many and could easily be combined with Detoxamin with the correct medical supervision (*Bruce, Roberts*). The dose is usually 1 oz. (1/2 of a bottle) in cranberry or other juice 2-3 times a week. There will be more about these great advances in self-chelation in upcoming *Total Wellness* issues as we finish evaluating/confirming their merits.

I'll remind you again, since this is often overlooked: If you find you still have, say too much mercury on board after many months, you may need to switch to Chemet or Captomer for a while. These are made of DMSA, a chemical that is better at removing mercury. Your physician should guide you with these more precise decisions after you have made a significant dent in your total heavy metals and other foreign chemical loads. Detoxamin is the best start.

Far Infrared Fountain of Youth

Detoxamin combined with your **Far Infrared Sauna Protocol** is what I consider the fountain of youth. As I showed in *Detoxify or Die*, the accumulation of unwanted chemicals starting when we were still in the uterus progresses throughout life and is a major cause of deterioration and disease. It makes great sense to get these chemicals out of the body and put the body back at a level that we had 20 or 30 years ago. The far infrared sauna is the best way I know of for getting rid of the majority of foreign chemicals that we slowly tank up on starting when we were still in the uterus. These are a fundamental cause of all disease, and especially of high blood pressure. And as I showed in *Detoxify or Die*, it is the only type of sauna proven in medical studies done at the famed Mayo Clinic and elsewhere to be safe even for delicate heart patients and patients with congestive heart failure. Normally any extra heat, much less a sauna would be contraindicated for delicate congestive heart failure patients.

You may recall that heart patients are notoriously sensitive to high heat, and are the first to die during heat waves. So a sauna is the last place you would put them. But because of its special low temperature combined with the healing energies of far infrared technology, not only did end-stage congestive heart failure patients tolerate the far infrared sauna, but they reversed their congestive heart failure after their cardiologists at the Mayo Clinic had exhausted everything medicine has to offer. These patients were at the end of their ropes, yet the far infrared sauna's special low heat protocol allowed them to drop medications as their blood pressures corrected, and their ejection fractions (a measure of the heart getting stronger) and other parameters improved. The far infrared sauna protocol is the only proven technology safe for heart patients while able to get unwanted chemicals out and reverse heart and other diseases for which medicine is stumped. (See *Detoxify or Die* for more details).

The cardiovascular system of heart and blood vessels is particularly vulnerable, for example, on days of high pollution. Inhalation of highway exhaust, factory exhausts, and incinerators have dramatically cut down the protective chemicals in the lining of blood vessels (endothelin-1 and angiotensin-converting enzyme mRNA) by as much as 60%. What does this do? Paralyze the ability of your silver lining to cause dilatation or expansion of the blood vessel, plus nudges the chemistry that encourages clots and plaque build-up inside vessels (*Nurkiewicz*). High pollutant exposures have already been proven to accelerate aging and arteriosclerosis as well as increase inflammation and plaque inside vessels. That is why it is important to also have a good air purifier in your car. You should get one (**E.L. Foust Co.**, 1-800-ELFOUST) that plugs right into the cigarette lighter (finally a good use for it). You know from *Detoxify or Die* that one of the easiest ways we get 500 rats with cancer for experiments is to give them a single dose of everyday common pollutants, including diesel and other vehicle emission exhausts. And clearly diesel exhaust contributes to lung cancer, allergies, and a host of other maladies that are merely treated as drug deficiencies. As the world gets more complicated and dangerous fortunately we still have some pretty simple and easy remedies that are unparalleled. Your Detox Cocktail and the **Far Infrared Sauna** can boost your detoxification of this daily onslaught of chemicals and accelerate you're getting rid of them before they accumulate to cause of disease.

Obviously if you have resistant high blood pressure, or if you have any other disease that you would like to reverse, or if you just plain want to be healthier and improve your athletic prowess and longevity, the **Far infrared Sauna** is a must as far as I'm concerned. And I haven't even given you half the benefits. For example, you can do it at home and you can get work accomplished while you are in it, so there is no lost time. It's a win-win situation for healing the impossible and boosting longevity if ever there was.

But there is a limit to how much you can sweat out in your far infrared sauna. Since it is the only way out of the body for some of the nastiest chemicals like the pesticides, plasticizers or phthalates, and volatile organic hydrocarbons, it makes sense to get as much mileage as we can out of this protocol and reserve use of the EDTA for the heavy metals. For in reality many people are far too sick to wait for years and years for their body to finally start get rid of the heavy metals as well with a sauna. They're just too loaded to be able to sweat all that out in time to save their lives. It makes more sense to use multiple avenues to speed up detoxifying the body, and these two (the Far Infrared Sauna and Detoxamin) are very harmonious. But I would strongly urge physician supervision and especially periodic monitoring of your loss of the good minerals.

The majority of chemicals stored in the body fat cannot be chelated like the heavy metals can. The far infrared sauna is the only proven way out of the body that is even safe for the ailing heart. For example, as I showed in *Detoxify or Die*, U.S. government EPA studies show that 100% of us have stored levels of carcinogenic PCBs in us. These man-made chemicals that are unavoidable and everywhere in our air, food, and water damage the ability to properly metabolize cholesterol, so we have high triglycerides and high cholesterol (*Hennig*). They damage the D5D and D6D desaturace enzymes so that we cannot properly convert the oils that we eat to the safe forms that protect our arteries. PCBs also turn on the chemistry of inflammation that leads not only to Mr. ED, endothelial dysfunction the precursor to high blood pressure and organ damage, but also to the chemistry that turns on arteriosclerosis and many other diseases (*Hennig*). The only proven heart-healthy way out of the body that I know is with the far infrared sauna.

So here you have it. For many of you, taking a few months to detoxify your heavy metals may be all you need to permanently cure your high blood pressure. For others it will take much longer or they may need to incorporate several of the other protocols that are in this book. Meanwhile, as you make your body healthier, don't be surprised when many other symptoms improve as well. Those are the "side effects" of natural medicine. Many things improve at once.

But your results will be commensurate with your knowledge and dedication. In *The E. I. Syndrome* you will learn about the importance of reducing the total load of chemical pollutants. Clearly little things mean a lot. For example, you may take for granted the harmlessness of your morning aftershave. But did you know that the chemicals that make up these fragrances are absorbed right through the skin and lungs to stockpile in the fat? (*Luckenbach*) Once in the body, their sneaky destruction of health begins. They promote the chemistry of cancer in the body by multiple mechanisms. But you don't have to wait years before you get a cancer to feel their secret effects. They add to the total hidden load of chemicals so that once ostensibly low or safe levels of chemical exposures now become toxic. They sensitize the system, leading to intolerance or toxicity from things that previously didn't bother you. And they allow chemicals to penetrate into your cells that previously could not get inside to do their damage. Likewise, the phthalates (plastizers), for example, in nail polish, hair spray and other cosmetics and toiletries (*Barrett*) silently damage the basic chemistry of the body ushering in any disease possible.

Caveats: There are lots of things to look out for, for example, if you start itching all over or having skin rashes, headaches, or unusual symptoms, stop your program to see if they go away. Sometimes heavy metals and other chemicals come out too fast, faster than your body can deal with them. Hence, symptoms are produced. Doing your **Detox Cocktail** and **Detox Enema** speeds up their elimination (also described more in *Detoxify or Die*). Obviously you should stop any chelation and sauna for a few days or weeks while your body catches up. Or you can mobilize heavy metals from your bones only to deposit them in other organs like the brain if you are not capable of getting rid of them completely at the time of mobilization from storage with your chelator.

Likewise if you feel really exhausted or wiped out, you probably are not keeping up with your mineral replenishment and you really should get the **RBC Mineral Panel** (MetaMetrix) to determine what you have become deficient in. Of course, the best bargain is the **ION Panel** which includes your fatty acids, amino acids, vitamins, and organic acids as well as the minerals and RBC heavy metals.

The Plasticizer Plague

In case you never heard of plasticizers (or phthalates as referred to in the biochemistry literature), they are the heaviest pollutants in the human body. They are over 1000 fold to one million times higher than anything else that has been found in EPA studies, including pesticides, volatile organic hydrocarbons from auto exhaust for example, and even heavy metals. And they do enormous damage, including create cancer (*Mastrangelo*).

Tufts University researchers showed that plasticizers actually migrate from plastic film (Saran Wrap™), Styrofoam trays, plastic bottles and other plastic containers directly into the foods that they are supposedly protecting. And once we eat these foods the plastics (phthalates) get stuck in our bodies' cells and cause enormous damage. They steadily accumulate because we don't always have enough detoxification capability to get rid of our everyday load.

Even some medications are a source of plasticizers (*Hauser*):
- Enteric coatings of pills, e.g. Asacol (the classic Rx for colitis) is coated with methacrylic acid copolymer B, and dermal adhesives like estrogen and testosterone patches also put plasticizers in the body

- IV tubing and bags, plus dialysis machines and IV chelation boost body levels.

As well, we get a dose of phthalates or plasticizers from body lotions and gels, shampoos, deodorants, adhesives, building materials, school/business supplies, PVC (water) pipes, furnishings, auto interiors, solvents, plastics, glues, lubricants, insect repellants, detergents, toys, and foods. For plastics serve many purposes: plastics hold color and scent plus plasticizers provide flexibility to materials.

Let's look a little closer at the sources of life-damaging plastics in our bodies, which we absorb right through the skin from our home and business environments. Where do they leach and outgas from? Everywhere. Anything polyvinyl, styrene, PVC, plastic, acrylic, or synthetic, from our clothes, shoes and textiles, and much more. So this includes everything from floor tiles, carpet backing and the adhesives to glue them down, to paints, wallpaper, furnishings, wood finishes, pesticides, detergents, ceiling tiles, office supplies, books, appliances, TVs, computers, etc. (*Silva*). Plastics have us covered in our air, food and water.

Once inside the body we steadily tank up on them. We were never designed for such an enormous daily onslaught. We just frankly cannot detoxify it all in one day, which is why they are in everyone (*Silva*). Unfortunately even babies are born with high levels if their mother had an IV at delivery or drank sodas or water out of a plastic bottle.

In the body, plastics make a beeline for little organelles inside cells called peroxisomes and for the genetic receptors that govern the peroxisomes, called PPAR (peroxisome proliferator-activated receptors). In essence, they then damage the chemistry that controls all of our fatty acids, glucose, triglycerides, beta-oxidation of fats and phospholipids or lipid homeostasis; they govern inflammation, immunity, the cell cycle, and much more. In essence they damage the very organelles through which fatty acids control genes for not only healthy blood vessels, but the heart, all body cell membranes, hormone receptors, cancer cytokines, and much more. Without making molecular biochemists out of you, suffice to say that once these unavoidably ubiquitous plastics make their way into the body (and no U.S. humans have been found who do not have them), they damage every aspect of crucial cell function.

As long as they are silently present, they make it impossible for many people to heal. Meanwhile they can silently damage the thyroid and damage other hormones like testosterone, or adrenal stress hormones, making it impossible to lose weight or regain energy, as they accelerate cancers as well as arteriosclerosis and high blood pressure (*Bell, Kliewer, Chinetti, Kim, Lapinskas, Brucker*).

If that were not enough, the mean daily intake of damaging cadmium is 0.3 mcg/l., while the mean daily organophosphate pesticide intake is 2.55 mcg/l. Compare that with the mean daily phthalate intake (of only *one* of several phthalate esters in the human body) of **176 mcg /l.** a day. This is over 1000 times higher than any other pollutant (Silva). In fact, the average **total daily phthalate intake is over 3 mg (3000 mcg), ten thousand times more** than deadly cadmium. That is why plastics are over a million times more plentiful in the human body than any other pollutant. With a half-life of 18 hours we don't get rid of it all each day. So we slowly poison ourselves until we one day awaken with a disease. The symptoms get a label, then we are sentenced to lifelong drugs. They secretly stall any attempt at getting well as they silently screw up the chemistry of every cell.

Reducing Plastics, As Easy As 1,2,3

When you get your 3 grams of phthalates today, what are you going to do to begin to get rid of it? First have your doctor measure your fatty acids, for when plastics poison the peroxisomes they cause blocks that lead to abnormal accumulations of fatty acids. High levels of arachidic, lignoceric, behenic, and hexacosanoic with mysteriously low levels of docosahexaenoic acid (DHA) are diagnostic of them. Then it gets serious, because the number one fatty acid in the brain and eye (DHA) is poisoned and nobody knows it. But it's completely repairable. And of course DHA is crucial for healthy vasculature (references in *TW* 2005).

So how do you get rid of plastics? It's as easy as 1, 2, 3:
1. Since they are detoxified primarily through glucuronidation (*Silva*), you can begin by taking **IndolPlex** and **Calcium D-Glucarate**, each 2 twice a day.
2. Also to rev up glucuronidation, the pathway the body uses to detoxify your daily plastics, have 2 or more servings of Brassica or cruciferous vegetables a day. These include cabbage, broccoli, Brussels sprouts, cauliflower, radishes, mizuna, watercress, arugula, turnips, collard greens, kale, rutabaga, and more. So what's so hard about a cabbage salad at lunch and some broccoli or collard greens at dinner? Or broccoli soup?
3. The only way I know of to get phthalates out is with your **Far Infrared Sauna.**

Considering the level of plastics we are exposed to daily in our air, food and water, if you ask me, we had better do all three for the 21st century plastic plague. Oh, and did I forget to mention a fourth solution? Vote with your shopping cart and try to avoid foods in plastic. Hey, if you think it's too hard, just think of all the majority of folks who don't even know that their symptoms are curable. At least you have a multitude of healing options.

Heavy Metals and Plastic Pollutants Are Just the Tip of the Iceberg

Even though I have concentrated on two of the nastiest pollutant categories, heavy metals and phthalates, we have by no means covered the spectrum. For example, just driving through traffic or going outside on a day of increased air pollution can raise your blood pressure, increase cardiovascular deaths, and change your heart's response to its own autonomic nervous system, called heart rate variability (*Pope, Peters, Grassi, Noll*). In other words, huge numbers of pollutants surround us from too many sources and they are only going to increase, making lifelong detoxification a priority. And, as one tiny example, when we deplete our own natural glutathione in the daily overwork of our detoxification chemistry, it causes high blood pressure (*Vaziri*): one more reason why you need your daily detox cocktail that you learned about in Chapter II.

You have done a great job. Let's go to the next chapter to see what else can normalize your blood pressure.

Product Sources:

- Far Infrared Sauna, High Tech Health, 1-800-7 94-5355
- Nutrient/Toxic Elements 24-hour urine, MetaMetrix, 1-800-221-4640
- RBC Mineral Panel, MetaMetrix, 1-800-221-4640
- ION Panel, MetaMetrix, 1-800-221-4640
- Castor Oil, prlabs.com, 1-800-370-3447
- Detoxamin, detoxamin.com, 1-877-656-4553
- NAC, jarrow.com, 1-800-726-0886
- Zinc Balance, jarrow.com, 1-800-726-0886
- BioSil, jarrow.com, 1-800-726-0886
- Cod Liver Oil, carlsonlabs.com, 1-800-323-4141
- Super 2 Daily, carlsonlabs.com, 1-800-323-4141
- B-Complete-100, carlsonlabs.com, 1-800-323-4141
- E-Gems Elite, carlsonlabs.com, 1-800-323-4141
- Chelated Manganese 20 mg, carlsonlabs.com, 1-800-323-4141
- Chelated Zinc 30 mg, carlsonlabs.com, 1-800-323-4141
- Selenium 200 mcg, carlsonlabs.com, 1-800-323-4141
- Chelated Chromium 200 mcg, carlsonlabs.com, 1-800-323-4141
- Moly B, carlsonlabs.com, 1-800-323-4141
- Liquid Multiple Minerals, carlsonlabs.com, 1-800-323-4141
- PhosChol 900, nutrasol.com, 1-800-364-4416
- IntraMin, druckerlabs.com, 1-972-881-2344
- Iodoral, Belmar Pharmacy, 1-303-763-5533
- Cogimax, Optimox, 1-800-223-1601.
- Boron, Pure Encapsulations, 1-800-753-2277
- Glycine, Taurine 1000 mg, Pain & Stress Center, 1-800-669-CALM
- Thisilyn, Bio-Tech, 1-800-345-1199
- IndolPlex (Integrative Therapeutics) NEEDS, 1-800-634-1380
- Calcium D-glucarate, (Integrative Therapeutics) NEEDS, 1-800-324-1380
- L-Arginine Powder, Carlson, 1-800-323-4141

Chelation Options:

- **Detoxamin,** microzyme@mindpring.com, 1-877 656-4553
- Medicardium, Bio Botanical, 1-800-775-4140
- DetoxMax Plus, bioimmune.com, 1-888-663-8844
- Captomer (Thorne 1-800-228-1966) NEEDS 1-800-846-6687
- Chemet, Rx any pharmacy
- Detox Cocktail detailed in Chapter II
- Magnesium sources detailed in Chapter I

References:

Sorensen N, Prenatal metal mercury exposure as a cardiovascular risk factor at seven years of age, *Epidemiology*, 10; 4:370-75, July 1999

Salonen JT, *Circulation* 91; 3: 6 45-55, February 1, 1995

Pottinger M, Stecklow S, Fialka JJ, Invisible export: A hidden cost of China's growth: mercury migration. Turning to coal, nation sends toxic metal around globe; buildup in the Great Lakes, *Wall Street J*, A-1, A8, Dec. 17, 2004

Eig J, Christmas embargo: A mom bans China from under the tree, *Wall Street Journal*, A1, A5, Dec. 24, 2004

Grandjean P, Jacobson IA, Jorgensen PJ, Chronic lead poisoning treated with demercaptosuccinic acid, *Pharmacol Toxicol*, 68; 4:266-69, 1991

Lee B, Schwartz BS, Stewart W, Ahn K, Provocative chelation with DMSA and EDTA; evidence for differential access to lead storage sites, *Occupation Environ Med*, 52:13-19, 1995

Aaseth J, et al, Treatment of mercury and lead poisonings with demercaptosuccinic acid and sodium dimercaptopropane sulfate, *Analyst*, 120:853-54, 1995

Smith D, Bayer L, Strupp B, Efficacy of succimer chelation for reducing brain lead levels in a rodent model, *Environ Res*, 78: 168-76, 1998

Aposhian HV, Maiorino RM, Aposhian MM, et al, Mobilization of heavy metals by newer, therapeutically useful chelating agents, *Toxicol*, 97:23-38, 1995

Bemis JC, Seegal RF, Polychlorinated biphenyls and methylmercury alter intracellular calcium concentrations in rats cerebellar granule cells, *Neurotox*, 21; 6:1123-1134, 2000

Guallar E, Sanz-Gallaardo M, Frans J, et al, Mercury, fish oils, and risk of myocardial infarction, *New Engl J Med*, 347; 22:1747-54, Nov. 28, 2002

Lustberg M, Silbergeld E, Blood lead levels and mortality, *Arch Intern Med*, 162: 2443-49, Nov. 25, 2002

Patrick L, Mercury toxicity and antioxidants: Part I: Role of glutathione and alpha-lipoic acid in the treatment of mercury toxicity, *Alt Med Rev*, 7; 6:456-71, 2002

Burmaster GE, The new pollution-groundwater contamination. *Environment* 24: 7-13, 33-36, 1982

Dyksen JE, Hess AF, Alternatives for controlling organics in groundwater supplies, *J Am Water Works Assoc* 74: 394-403, 1982

Page JW, Comparison of groundwater and surface water for patterns and levels of contamination by toxic substances. *Environ Sci Technol* 15: 1475-81, 1981

Jones DP, Chemical levels detected in people alarm scientists, *LA Times*, A14, Aug. 21, 2000

(CDC) Centers for Disease Control and Prevention, *National Report on Human Exposure to Environmental Chemicals*, NCEH publication No. 01-0164, CDC, National Center for Environmental Health, Atlanta GA, 1-866-690-6052, March 2001

Ross GL, Rogan WJ, Collignon P, et al, The DDT question. *Lancet*, 356:1189-91, 2000

Castle L, Mercer AJ, Startin JR, et al, Migration from plasticized films into foods: 3. Migration of phthalate, sebacate, citrate and phosphate esters from films used for retail food packaging. *Food Addit Contam* 5; 1: 9-20, 1988

Eriksson P, Jakobsson E, Fredriksson A, Brominated flame retardants: A novel class of developmental neurotoxicants in our environment? *Environ Health Persp* 109; 9: 903-08 Sept 2001

Muckle G, Ayotte P, Jacobson JL, et al, Determinants of polychlorinated biphenyls and methylmercury exposure in Inuit women of childbearing age, *Environ Health Persp* 109; 9: 957-64, Sept 2001

Mielke HW, Powell ET, Mielke PW, et al, Multiple metal contamination from housepaints: Consequences of power sanding and paint scraping in New Orleans, *Environ Health Persp* 109; 9: 9 3-78, Sept 2001

Kadiislka RI, Dikalova A, Thurman RG, et al, Phthalate rapidly increases production of reactive oxygen species *in vivo*: role of Kupffer cells, *Mol Pharmacol*, 59; 4: 744-50, Apr 2001

Vaziri ND, et al, Induction of oxidative stress by glutathione depletion causes severe hypertension in normal rats, *Hypertension* 36: 142-146, 2000

Bell FP, Effects of phthalate esters on lipid metabolism in various tissues, cells and organelles in mammals, *Environ Health Persp* 45: 41-50, 1982

War and JR, et Al, Phthalate esters as peroxisome proliferator carcinogens, *Environ Health Persp*, 45: 35-40, 1982

133

Rock G, et al, Hypotension and cardiac arrest in rats after infusion of mono (2-ethylhexyl) phthalate (MEHP), a contaminant in stored blood, *New Engl J Med,* 316; 19: 148-49, May 7, 1987

Sterzl I, et al, Mercury and nickel allergy: risk factors in fatigue and autoimmunity, *Neuro-endocrinology Letters* 20: 221-28, 1999

Unger M. Olsen J, Organochlorine compounds in the adipose tissue of deceased people with and without cancer, *Environ Res* 23: 257-63, 1980

Kilburn KH, Warsaw RH, Shields MG, Neurobehavioral dysfunction in firemen exposed to polychlorinated biphenyls (PCBs): Possible improvement after detoxification, *Arch Environ Health,* 44; 6:345-350, 1989

Schnare DW, Ben M, Shields MG, Body burden reductions of PCBs, PBBs and chlorinated pesticides in human subjects *Ambio,* 13;5-6:378-80, 1984

Roehm DC, Effects of a program of sauna baths and megavitamins on adipose DDE and PCBs and on clearing of symptoms of agent orange (Dioxin) toxicity, *Clin Res* 31; 2:243A, 1983

Rea W. J., Pan Y, Fenyves, EJ, et al. Reduction of chemical sensitivity by means of heat de-puration, physical therapy and nutritional supplementation in a controlled environment, *J Nutr Environ Med,* 7; 2: 141-48, 1996

Hubbard LR, *Clear Body Clear Mind,* Bridge Publications, 4751 Fountain Avenue, Los Angeles CA 90029, 1990, 1-888-514-8788

Muckle G, Ayotte P, Jacobson JL, et al, Prenatal exposure of the Northern Quebec Inuit infants to environmental contaminants, *Environ Health Persp,* 109; 12: 1291-1299, Dec 2001

Persky V, Turyk M, Great Lakes Consortium, et al, The effects of PCB exposure and fish consumption on endogenous hormones, *Environ Health Persp,* 109; 12:1275-1283, Dec 2001

Schantz SL, Widholm JJ, Cognitive effects of endocrine-disrupting chemicals in animals, *Environ Health Persp,* 109; 12:. 1197-1206, Dec 2001

Imamura M, Biro S, Kihara T, Tei C, et al, Repeated thermal therapy improves impaired vascular endothelial functions in-patients with coronary risk factors, *J Am Coll Cardiol,* 38; 4: 1083-1087, 2001

Ikeda Y, Biro S, Kamogawa Y, et al, Repeated thermal therapy upregulates arterial endothelial nitric oxide synthase expression in Syrian golden hamsters, *Jpn Circul J,* 65: 434-38, 2001

Schwartz J, Otto D, Lead and minor hearing impairment, *Arch Environ Health* 46: 300-3005, 1991

Schwartz J, Low-level lead exposure and children's IQ: a meta-analysis and search for a threshold, *Environ Res* 65: 42-55, 1994

Lanphear BP, Dietrich KN, Auinger P, Cox C, Cognitive deficits associated with blood lead levels <10ug/dl in U.S. children and adults, *Public Health Rep*, 115: 521-529, 2000

Zanobetti A, Schwartz J, Dockery DW, Airborne particles are a risk factor for hospital admissions for heart and lung disease, *Environ Health Persp*, 108: 1071-77, 2000

Laden F, Neas LM, Dockery DW, Schwartz J, Association of fine particulate matter from different sources with daily mortality in six U.S. cities, *Environ Health Persp*, 108: 941-947, 2000

Janssen NAH, Schwartz J, Zanobetti A, Suh HH, Air conditioning and source-specific particles as modifiers of the effect of PM10 on hospital admissions for heart and lung disease, *Environ Health Persp*, 110; 1:43-49, 2002

Wong CM, Atkinson RW, Lam TH, et al, A tale of two cities: Effects of air pollution on hospital admissions in Hong Kong and London compared, *Environ Health Persp*, 110; 1: 67-77, 2002

Wolff MS, Anderson HA, Seilikoff IJ, Human tissue burdens of halogenated aromatic chemicals in Michigan, *J Am Med Assoc*, 247; 15: 2112-16, 1982

Martineau D, Lemberger K, Mikaelian I, et al, Cancer in wildlife, a case study: Beluga from the St. Lawrence estuary, Quebec, Canada, *Environ Health Persp*, 110; 3: 285-92, Mar 2002

Theriault GP, Tremblay CG, Armstrong BG, Risk of ischemic heart disease among the primary aluminum production workers, *Am J Indust Med* 13: 659-66, 1988

Bond JA, Gown AM, Juchau MR, et al, Further investigations of the capacity of polynuclear aromatic hydrocarbons to elicit atherosclerotic lesions, *J Toxicol Environ Health* 7: 327-35, 1981

Levine RJ , Andjelkovich DA, Kersteter SL, et al, Heart disease in workers exposed to dinitrotoluene, *J Occup Med* 28: 8 11-16, 1986

Atkins E. H., Baker EL, Exacerbation of coronary artery disease by occupational carbon monoxide exposure: a report of two fatalities and a review of the literature, *Am J Indust Med* , 7: 73-79, 1985

Aronow WS, Stemmer EA, Isbell MW, Effect of carbon monoxide exposure on intermittent claudication, *Circulation* 249: 415-17, 1974

Kesteloot H, Roeland J, Joosens JV, et al, An inquery into the role of cobalt in the heart disease are chronic beer drinkers, *Circulation* 37: 854-64, 1968

Alexander CS, Cobalt and the heart, *Ann Intern Med* 70: 411-13, 1969

Goldsmith S, Arsenic-induced atypical ventricular tachycardia, *New Engl J Med* 303: 1096-98, 1980

Klein T. S., Myocardial changes in lead poisoning, *Am J Dis Child* 99: 48, 1960

Myerson RM, Eisenhauler JH, Atrioventricular conduction defects in lead poisoning, *Am J Cardiol* 11: 409-12, 1963

Asokan SK, Experimental lead cardiomyopathy: myocardial structural changes in rats given small amounts of lead. *J Lab Clin Med* 84: 20-25, 1974

Williams BJ, Hejtmancik MR, Abreu M, Cardiac effects of lead. *Fed Proceed* 42: 2989-93,1983

Mee AS, Wright PL, Congestive (dilated) cardiomyopathy in association with solvent abuse, *J Roy Soc Med* 73: 671-72, 1980

McLeod AA, Marjot R, Jackson G., et al, Chronic cardiac toxicity after inhalation of 1, 1,1-trichloroethane, *Brit Med J* 294: 728-29, 1987

Wiseman MN, Banim S, "Blue sniffer's" heart? *Brit Med J*, 294: 739, 1987

Right MS, Strobl DJ, 1, 1,1-trichloroethane cardiac toxicity: report of a case, *J Am Ostropath Assoc* 84: 285-88, 1984

Speizer FE, Wegman DH, Ramirez A, Palpitation rates associated with fluorocarbon exposure in a hospital setting, *New Engl J Med*, 292: 624-26, 1975

Antti-Poika N, Heikkila J, Saarinen L, Cardiac arrhythmias during occupational exposure to fluoridated hydrocarbons, *Brit J Indust Med* 47: 1 38-40, 1990

Edling C, Ohlson CG, Soderholm B, et al, Cardiac arrhythmia in refrigerator repairman exposed to fluorocarbons, *Brit J Indust Med*, 47: 207-12, 1990

Kobayshi S, Hutchenon DE, Regan J, Cardiopulmonary toxicity of tetrachloroethylene, *J Toxicol Environ Health* 10:23-30, 1982

Ludomirshy A, Klein HO, Sarelli P, et al, Q-T prolongation and polymorphous ("torsade de pointes") ventricular arrhythmias associated with or organophosphorus insecticide poisoning, *Am J Cardiol* 49: 1654-58, 1982

Sharp DS, Becker CE, Smithey AH, Chronic low-level lead exposure: its role in the pathogens is of hypertension, *Med Toxicol* 2: 210-32, 1987

Schroeder H. A., Cadmium, chromium, and cardiovascular disease, *Circulation* 35: 575-82, 1967

Kihara T, Biro S, Imamura M, Yoshifuku S, Takasaki K, Ikeda Y, Tei C, et al, Repeated sauna treatment improves the vascular endothelial and cardiac function in patients with chronic heart failure, *J Am Coll Cardiol*, 39; 5:754-9, Mar 2002

Tei C, Horikiri Y, Park JC, et al, Acute hemodynamic improvement by thermal vasodilatation in congestive heart failure, *Circulation* 91: 2582-90, 1995

Tei C, Tanaka N, Thermal vasodilatation as a treatment of congestive heart failure: a novel approach, *J Cardiol* 27: 29-30, 1996

Henderson GL, Wilson BK, Excretion of methadone and metabolites in human sweat, *Res Comm Chem Pathol Pharmacol* 5; 1: 1-8, Jan 1973

Vree TB, Muskens AT, VanRosum JM, Excretion of amphetamines in human sweat, *Arch Intern Pharmacodyn* 199: 311-17, 1972

Udagawa Y, Nagasawa H, Kiyokawa S, Inhibition by whole-body hyperthermia with far-infrared rays of the growth of spontaneous mammary tumors in mice, *Anticancer Res* 19: 4125-30, 1999

Kreiss K, Zack MM, Jones BT, et al, Association of blood pressure and polychlorinated biphenyl levels, *J Am Med Assoc*, 245: 2505-09, 1981

Chisholm JJ, Safety and efficacy of meso-2,3-dimercaptosuccinic acid (DMSA) in children with elevated blood lead concentrations, *J Toxicol Clin Toxicol* 38:365-375, 2000

Cotton P, "Best data yet" state air pollution kills below levels currently considered safe, *J Am Med Assoc* 269; 24: 3087-8, June 23, 1993

Gregus A, Stein AF, Varga R, Klaasen CD, Effect of lipoic acid in the biliary excretion of glutathione and metals, *Toxicol Appl Pharmacol*, 114; 1:88-96, 1992

Kopp SJ, Barron JT, Tow JP, Cardiovascular actions of lead and relationship to hypertension: a review, *Environ Health Perspect*, 78:91-99, 1988

Moller L, Kristensen T, Blood lead as a cardiovascular risk factor, *Am J Epidemiol* 136:1091-1100, 1992

Chai SS, Webb RC, Effects of lead on vascular reactivity, *Environ Health Perspect*, 78:85-89, 1988

Schwartz J. Lead, blood pressure, and cardiovascular disease in men, *Arch Environ Health*, 50:31-37, 1995

Cheng Y, Schwartz J, Hu H, et al, Bone lead and blood lead levels in relation to baseline blood pressure and the prospective development of hypertension, *Am J Epidemiol*, 153:164-71, 2001

Salonen JT, Seppanen K, Nyyssonen K, et al, Intake of mercury from fish, lipid peroxidation, and the risk of myocardial infarction and coronary, cardiovascular, and any death in eastern Finnish men, *Circulation*, 91:645-55, 1995

Rogers SA, *Detoxify Or Die*, prestigpublishing.com or 1-800-846-6687

Kramer JA, Pettit SD, Afshari CA, et al, Overview of the application of transcription profiling using selected nephrotoxicants for toxicology assessment, *Environ Health Persp*, 112: 460-464, 2004

Andoh TF, Gardner MP, Bennett WM, Protective effects of dietary L-arginine supplementation on chronic cyclosporine nephrotoxicity. *Transplantation* 64: 12 36-40, 1997

137

Hauser R, et al, Medications as a source of human exposure to phthalates, *Environ Health Persp*, 112; 6:751-53, 2004

Silva MJ, Barr DB, Calafat AM, et al, Urinary levels of seven phthalate metabolites in the U.S. population from the National Health and Nutrition Examination Survey (NHANES) 1999-2000, *Env Health Perspect* 112: 331-38, 2004

Bruce E, Chouinard RA, Tall AR, Plasma lipid transfer proteins, high-density lipoproteins, and reverse cholesterol transport, *Annu Rev Nutr*, 18: 297-330, 1998

Wartman A, Lampe TL, McCann DS, Boyle AJ, Plaque reversal with Mg EDTA in experimental atherosclerosis: elastin and collagen metabolism. *J Atheroscler Res*, 7: 31-41, 1967

Roberts J, reference PowerPoint lectures given at many CME approved physician courses across the United States available from the company (1-877-656-4553)

Bell FP, Effects of phthalate esters on lipid metabolism in various tissues, cells and organelles in mammals, *Environ Health Persp* 45: 41-50, 1982

Kliewer SA, Fatty acids and eicosanoids regulate gene expression through direct interactions with PPAR, *Proc Nat Acad Sci* 94:4318-23, 1997

Chinetti G, et al, PPAR: nuclear receptors at the crossroads between lipid metabolism and inflammation, *Inflamm Res*, 49; 10:497-505, 2000

Kim SC, Hong JT, Yun YP, et al, Formation of 8-oxodeoxyguanosine in liver DNA and hepatic injury by peroxisome proliferator clofibrate and perfluorodecanoic acid in rats, *J Toxicol; Sci* 23; 2; 113-119, 1998

Lapinskas P, Corton C, Mechanisms of hepatocarcinogenic peroxisome proliferators, In: *Molecular Biology of the Toxic Response* (Puga A, Wallace KB, eds.). Philadelphia, Taylor & Francis, 219-254, 1999

Brucker DF, Effects of environmental synthetic chemicals on thyroid function, *Thyroid*, 8:827-56, 1998

Cranton E, Brecher A, *Bypassing Bypass*, Medex Publ, Troutdale VA, 1990
Halstead BW, *The Scientific Basis of EDTA Chelation Therapy*, Golden Quill Publ, Colton CA, 1979

ACAM courses: The American College for the Advancement of Medicine provides voluminous references in the syllabus for physicians attending courses, and they can be purchased separately, 1-800-532-3688.

Rosenman RH, Smith MK, The effect of certain chelating substances, salts of ethylenediamine-tetraacetic acid (EDTA), upon cholesterol metabolism in the rat. *J Clin. Invest.* 35:11-19, 1956

Blumer W. Calcium-disodium-EDTA treatment for cardiovascular symptoms. *Plzen Lek Sborn Suppl.* 62:157-159, 1990

138

Toyota H, Shibata S (Kyoto University). Supplementary studies on pharmacology of disodium ethylenediaminetetraacetate (EDTA salt). *Nippon Yakuriguku Zasshi.*52: 1-9, 1956

Uhl HSM, Brown HH, Zlatkis A, Zak, B, Myers GB, Boyle AJ. Effect of ethylenediaminetetraacetic acid (EDTA) on cholesterol metabolism in man. Preliminary report of effect of parenteral and oral administration of disodium and calcium salts. *Am J Clin Pathol.* 23:1226-1233, 1953

Oser BL, Oser M, Spencer HC, Safety evaluation studies of calcium EDTA. *Toxicol Appl Pharmacol.* 5:142-162,1963

Sidbury JB Jr., Bynum JC, Fetz LL, (US Public Health Serv.) Effect of chelating agent on urinary lead excretion. Comparison of oral and intravenous administration. *Proc Soc Exper Biol Med.* 82:226-228. (1444), 1953

Davidson L, Almgren A, Hurrell RF. Sodium iron EDTA (NaFe(III) EDTA) as a food fortificant does not influence absorption and urinary excretion of manganese in healthy adults. *J Nutr.* 128(7): 1139-1143,1998

Mariani B, Bisetti A, Romeo V, Blood-cholesterol-lowering action of the sodium salt of calciumethylenediaminetetraacetic acid. *Gazs Intern Med Chir.* 62:1812-1823, 1957. [Two g. daily of the drug, in 2 intravenous administrations, or (with a lower effect) by mouth or rectum, caused in humans a decrease of blood cholesterol, especially of its free fraction.]

Mitchell Jr PH, Schroeder HA. Depression of cholesterol levels in human plasma following ethylenediamine tetracetate and hydralazine. *J Chron Dis.* 2:520-533, 1955

Gordon GF, EDTA and chelation therapy: history and mechanisms of action - an update. *Clin. Pract. Altern. Med.* 2:36-45, 2001

Gordon: Dr. Gary Gordon has the worlds' largest compilation of references on oral EDTA, also has designed oral chelation products: Longevity Plus 1-800-580-PLUS

Gordon G. Oral chelation for improved heart function. *Life Enhancement*, 7-15, Apr 1997

Olszewer E, Sabbag FC, Carter JP, A pilot double-blind study of sodium-magnesium EDTA in peripheral vascular disease, *J Nat Med Assoc*, 82; 3:173-77, 1990

Olszewer E, Carter JP, EDTA chelation therapy in chronic degenerative disease, *Med Hypoth*, 27:41-49, 1988

Rudolph CJ, McDonagh EW, Barber RK, A nonsurgical approach to obstructive carotid stenosis using EDTA chelation, *J Advance Med*, 4; 3:157-66, fall 1991

Chappell LT, Stahl JP, The correlation between EDTA chelation therapy and improvement in cardiovascular function: a meta-analysis, *J Advance Med*, 6; 3:133-60, fall 1993

Kindness G, Frackelton JP, Effect of ethylene diamine tetraacetic acid (EDTA) on platelet aggregation in human blood, *J Advance Med*, 2.4:519-29, winter 1989

Rudolph CJ, McDonagh EW, Effect of EDTA chelation and supportive multivitamine trace mineral supplementation on carotid circulation,: case report, *J Advance Med*, 3;1:5-11, spring 1990

Gooneratne R, Olkowski A, Lead toxicity chelation therapy: new findings, *J Advance Med*, 6; 4:225-225-31, winter 1993

Schroeder HA, A practical method for the reduction of plasma cholesterol in man, *J Chron Dis*, 4; 5:461- 68, Nov 1956

Riordan HD, EDTA chelation/hypertension study, *J Orthomol Med*, 4; 2:91-95, 1989

Yechiel E, Barenholz Y, Relationships between membrane lipid composition and biological properties of rat myocytes. Effects of aging and manipulation of lipid composition, *J Biol Chem*, 260; 16:9123-31, Aug. 5, 1985

Yechiel E, Henis YE, Barenholz Y, Aging of rat heart fibroblast: relationship between lipid composition, membrane organization and biological properties, *Biochim Biophys Acta*, 859; 1: 95-104, July 10, 1986

Yechiel E, Barenholz Y, Cultured heart cell reaggregates: a model for studying relationships between aging and lipid composition, *Biochim Biophys Acta*, 859; one: 105-9, July 10, 1986

Bar LK, Barenholz Y, Thompson TE, Effect of sphingomyelin composition on the phase structure of phosphatidylcholine-sphingomyelin bilayers, *Biochem*, 3; 9: 2507-16, Mar. 4, 1997

Samochowiec L, On the action of the sensual phospholipids in experimental atherosclerosis, page 211-26, in Peeters H,ed., *Phosphatidylcholine, Biochemical and Clinical Aspects of The Essential Phospholipids*, Springer-Verlag,, NY 1976

Howard AN, Patelski J, Effect of EPA on the lipid metabolism of the arterial wall and other tissues, page 187-200, in Peeters H,ed., *Phosphatidylcholine, Biochemical and Clinical Aspects of The Essential Phospholipids*, Springer-Verlag,, NY 1976

Samochowiec L, Kadlubowsha D, Rozewicka L, Investigations in experimental atherosclerosis: part 1: The effects of phosphatidylcholine (EPL) on experimental atherosclerosis in white rats, *Atherosclerosis* 23: 305-17, 1976

Samochowiec L, Kadlubowsha D, Rozewicka L, Kuzna W, Szyska K, Investigations in experimental atherosclerosis: part 2: The effects of phosphatidylcholine (EPL) on experimental atherosclerotic changes in miniature pigs, *Atherosclerosis* 23: 319-31 1976

Stafford W. W., Day CE, Regression of atherosclerosis affected by intravenous phospholipid, *Artery*, 1: 106-114, 1975

Trachtman H, Del Pizzo R, Sturman JA, et al, Taurine lowers blood pressure in spontaneously hypertensive rat by a catecholamuine independent mechanism, *Am J Hypertens*, 2; 909-12, 1989

Nakagawa M, Takeda K, Sasaki S, et a., Antihypertensive effect of taurine on salt-induced hypertension, *Adv Exp Med Biol*, 359:197-206, 1994

Kohashi N, Okabayashi T, Katori R, et al, Decreased urinary taurine in essential hypertension, *Prog Clin Biol Res*, 125:73-87, 1983

Houston MC, The role of vascular biology, nutrition and nutraceuticals in the prevention and treatment of hypertension, *J Am Nutraceut Assoc*, suppl 1, Apr 2002

Pope CA III, Verrier RL, Kanner RE, etal, Heart rate variability associated with particulate air pollution, *Am Heart J*, 138:890-99, 1999

Peters A, et al, Increased plasma viscosity during air pollution episode: a link to mortality? *Lancet* 349:1582-87, 1997

Grassi G, Role of the sympathetic nervous system in human hypertension, *J Hypert* 161979-87, 1998

Noll G, et al, Role of sympathetic nervous system in hypertension, *Eur Heart J*, 19 (suppl F): F32-38, 1998

Silva MJ, Barr DB, Hodge CC, et al, Glucuronidation patterns of common urinary and serum monoester phthalate metabolites, *Arch Toxicol*, 77:561-7, 2003

Silva MJ, Barr DB, Calafat AM, et al, Urinary levels of seven phthalate metabolites in the U.S. population from the National Health and Nutrition Examination Survey (NHANES) 1999-2000, *Environ Health Perspect*, 112; 3:331-338, 2004

Bellinger DC, Stiles KM, Needleman HL, Low-level lead exposure, intelligence and academic achievement: a long-term follow-up study, *Pediatrics*, 90:855-61, 1992

Tsaih SW, Korrick Hu H, et al, Lead, diabetes, Hypertension, and renal function: the normative aging study, *Environ Health Perspect*, 112; 11:1178-82, 2004

Lin C, Kim R, Hu H, et al, Determinants of bone and blood lead levels among minorities living in the Boston area, *Environ Health Perspect*, 112; 11:1147-51, 2004

Mastrangelo G, Fedeli U, Matines D, et al, Increased risk of hepatocellular carcinoma and liver cirrhosis in vinyl chloride workers: Synergistic effect of occupational exposure with alcohol intake, *Environ Health Perspect*, 112; 11:1188-92, 2004

Nurkiewicz TR, Porter DW, Boegehold MA, et al., Particulate matter exposures impairs systemic microvascular endothelium-dependent dilatation, *Environ Health Persp*, 112; 13:1299-1306, 2004

Vaziri ND, Wang XQ, Oveisi F, Rad B, Induction of oxidative stress by glutathione depletion causes severe hypertension in normal rats, *Hypertension*, 36:142-46, 2000

Luckenbach T, Epel D, Nitromusk and polycyclic musk compounds as long-term inhibitors of cellular xenobiotic defense systems mediated by multidrug transporters, *Environ Health Perspect*, 113; 1:17-25, 2005

Barrett JR, The ugly side of beauty products, *Environ Health Perspect*, 113; 1:A24, 2005

Schafer JH, Glass TA, Schwartz BS, et al, Blood lead is a predictor of homocysteine levels in a population-based study of older adults, *Environ Health Persp*, 113; 1: 31-35, 2005

Homocysteine Collaboration, Homocysteine and risk of ischemic heart disease and stroke: a meta- analysis, *J Am Med Assoc*, 288: 2015-22, 2002

Rodrigo et al., Implications of oxidative stress and homocysteine in the pathophysiology of essential hypertension, *J Cardiovasc Pharmacol*, 42: 453-61, 2003

Nash D, et al., Blood lead, blood pressure, and hypertension in perimenopausal and post - menopausal women, *J Am Med Assoc*, 289:1523-32, 2003

Canfield RL, Henderson CR, Lanphear BP, et al, Intellectual impairment in children with blood lead concentrations below 10 mcg per dl, *New Engl J Med*, 348: 1517-26, 2003

Hennig B, Reiterer G, Robertson LW, et al, Dietary fat interacts with PCBs to induce changes in lipid metabolism in mice deficient in low-density lipoprotein receptor, *Environ Health Persp*, 113; 1: 83-87, 2005

P.S. If this chapter is too difficult for you now, concentrate on the remedies in the other chapters that are easier and more appealing to you. Plus you ideally want to assay and correct your **ION Panel** first to be sure your detoxification capability is maximized. You can always return to this if your body insists on being detoxified.

P.P.S. In *Detoxify or Die* is a 12-page letter that folks have used to convince their insurance companies to cover their far infrared saunas.

Chapter V

The Food Factor

The Celery Solution

I love the field of medicine. You can have a disease like hypertension that plagues over 68 million in the U.S. and the solutions can range from something incredibly simple to the complicated. Take celery. Celery can lower your blood pressure. It actually contains a God-designed phytochemicals like apigenin and 3-N butyl phthalide which can relax blood vessels, providing the benefits of calcium channel blockers without the proven brain shrinking that I've referenced for you in Chapter I, as well as diuretic effects and hormonal effects like lowering norepinephrine (*Le*).

How much do you need? **Four stalks of celery a day have been shown to significantly and safely lower blood pressure.** Please choose organic, available now in many conventional groceries. As well, the fiber is great for your gut and it will fill you up so you don't over-eat. You could make humus, or other bean or veggie dips to accompany it. What do you have to lose and what could be easier?

Remember Potassium?

It has been proven that potassium deficiency is a major cause of hypertension for many (*Barri, Taddei, Cappuccio, Follmann, Smith, Fotherby, Whelton, Khaw, MacGregor*). And correcting it likewise has cured many folks' blood pressure (*Whelton*). Clearly the best way to get good potassium levels is with a whole foods diet which I will outline, high in whole grains, beans, fruits, vegetables, nuts and seeds and other phyto-chemicals like green tea. And you recall from Chapter I that a major loss of potassium occurs with the first-line treatment for hypertension, diuretics. Also recall that you cannot maintain potassium levels at a normal range without the help of magnesium (*Altura, Wester, Classen*). Yet potassium and magnesium deficiencies alone or in combination are also potent causes of hypertension, acting either alone or in com-bination with other additional deficiencies. How intricately and precisely we are designed!

Clearly the best source of potassium is a whole foods diet: grains, greens and beans. That means real food that still has the life force in it. For example, you could sprout brown rice in a dish on the windowsill and grow a little rice plant. But if you put bleached instant rice or any boxed rice cereals there they would only rot and do not have half the nutri-tional value of the whole food.

But to get your mineral levels up higher, faster than with diet, you can start by adding supplements. If you have potassium deficiency on the RBC Minerals Panel (also part of the more complete test, ION Panel), you could temporar-ily take potassium in the form of **Complexed Potassium**. But because 99 mg is all the government will allow non-prescription, you may need 3-10 a day or even more. It makes more sense in the long run and for your overall per-manent good health to start with frequent carrot and other fresh vegetable juices several times a day while you perma-nently repair the damaged potassium channels in your cell membranes, as you learned in Chapters III and IV.

What is the most important aspect? (1) The oil change you learned about in Chapter III to repair the cell membrane that houses the potassium channels, and then (2) a detoxification program to get the phthalates (plasticizers) out of the peroxisomes (Chapter IV). For plastics poison the intracellular peroxisomes which govern the chemistry or composition of every cell membrane and its ion channels in the body. Many people are stranded forever with a specific illness or diagnosis and can never heal past a certain point until this stage is repaired. These coupled with your improved diet should rejuvenate and keep your potassium channels working great.

Is lack of potassium the cause of all high blood pressure? Absolutely not. In fact an even more common cause of high blood pressure is a deficiency in the other mineral that is also wasted by diuretics, magnesium. The leading cause of magnesium deficiency again is the processed foods diet. In fact government studies show that the average American diet only gives you 40% or less than half the magnesium you need in a day. Then other things like sweating, stress and anger, sugar, alcohol, medications, including diuretics again, accelerate the loss even further, resulting in not only higher pressure, but arrhythmias, angina, heart failure or sudden cardiac death (*Mountokalakis, Altura, Singh*). So by all means review Chapter I to make sure you are getting 400-600 mg of magnesium a day (and not the poorly absorbed oxide form).

Let's Do Lunch...7-11 or the Gas Station?

I'm utterly amazed at how many workers "dine" at the local 7-11 or gas station for breakfast and lunch. Cars and trucks are lined up, double parked, and waiting lines are intense.

But when I peek over their shoulders to see what these folks are eating, it was all processed dead foods, loaded with disease-producing trans fatty acids, MSG, pesticides, additives, and stripped of nutritional value. Hot dogs, pizza slices, gooey doughnuts, pre-made sandwiches of nitrate-laced cold cuts with large amounts of trans fatty acid mayonnaise, and large Cokes dominated the scene.

Whenever I have gone into a 7-11 to get a newspaper, a quick look around has confirmed there was absolutely no living food. I've never seen a solitary thing in there that I would eat. The closest to living food were some highly waxed apples I saw once!

Processed foods that come out of a bag, box, can, jar, or wrapper have a list of chemical additives and have been subjected to manufacturing processes that drop the original nutritional value by as much as 80%. Eating as close to nature as possible can boost the immune system's bug-fighting ability immensely, as well as lower blood pressure. But I know changing dietary habits is one of the most difficult things to do. So let's see how you could simply just improve breakfast and lunch, two out of three meals.

Whole Foods Diet

I've streamlined the live food diet for you so you can start to rejuvenate your body, since a whole foods diet is one of the most healing and/or preventive ways to eat for hypertension (*Maizes, Joshipura, Gillman, Pins*). For starters, use the birdseed cereal of soaked raw buckwheat grouts, sunflower seeds and almonds, adding kefir or organic yogurt and fruits of your choice (more details in *Detoxify or Die*). The **Natural**

Lifestyle catalog, 1-800-752-2775, is my favorite source for non-GMO organic whole grains, beans, seed, nuts and teas and much more. In fact they are one of the last few suppliers in the world that I know of to be dedicated to organic, non-genetically tampered with food.

Lunch could be a huge salad with unlimited raw vegetables of your choice. Don't forget great additions like avocado, almond slivers, cashews or walnuts, shiitake or portobello mushrooms, grated cheeses, gorgonzola, apple or pear slices, or sunflower seeds. Use your imagination. If you are afraid you still need more protein, add some hard boiled eggs or canned Alaskan wild salmon that has not been fed pink dye so that it looks artificially fresh (**Seafood Direct** catalog, 1-800-732-1836) or left over sliced organic chicken or non-farmed grilled salmon from dinner.

Your dressing should be a top-quality organic cold pressed oil of your choice, fresh lemon juice or rice wine or balsamic vinegar, fresh herbs like cilantro or basil, minced fresh garlic and even a little maple syrup if you need sweetening. Again use your imagination, but make sure that ingredients are top-quality. This can easily be prepared the night before (keep your dressing in a separate little jar) for carrying to work. Bring along 2-4 great fruits for dessert and your glass-bottled water. This makes a great start for transition to a more healthful change toward a special whole foods diet which has even been used to reverse cancers, after everything else has failed. *Macro Mellow* contains recipes and menus for whole foods cooking.

If you are on the road and salads are too messy for your lunchtime, bring along humus made at home from your own delicious organic spiced beans (see *Macro Mellow*) or buy it ready-made from the local health food store. A zip-lock baggy keeps a variety of vegetable sticks very fresh. Julienne carrots, celery, scallions, anise root, zucchini, cauliflower, radishes, and broccoli are just a few of the many healthful vegetables for your humus dip. Bring along a hunk of organic cheddar cheese if you like and some great raw cashews, pecans, raisins, dates or a tangerine for dessert.

Eating like this for just one month will convince you of the power of food. Getting off dead, devitalized processed foods and substituting whole foods that were recently alive (and have not been mangled and cooked to death in some factory) will energize your whole system. First of all, you will have easy non-smelly bowel movements shortly, since all that fiber is not only good for cleansing the bowel but helps heal the gut's immune system and is strongly anti-carcinogenic. If you cannot handle the fruits because of Candida, isn't it about time you got rid of your Candida? If your gut is too sensitive for all this fiber, likewise, heal it. Start with *No More Heartburn*, then go to *Detoxify or Die*. After all, time is of the essence and is wasting. Get on with your healing. On days when you are too tired to eat well, at least detoxify your gut while you possibly lower your blood pressure as many have with 1-3 tbs. of dried greens in the tasty form of Wakunaga's **Kyo-Green** (*Merchant*).

A Diet that Removes Plaque from Arteries

A macrobiotic diet is even more healing if whole foods are not to your liking or are too rough on your gut. I first became aware of the healing power of the macrobiotic diet when I witnessed multiple people who had healed end-stage

148

cancers, *after* medicine had given up on them. They had been given anywhere from 2-20 weeks to six months to live and survived beyond 22 years. You won't hear about this from the American Cancer Society and National Cancer Institute, in fact they recommend against it. There's no money in it.

Needless to say, if it's strong enough to reverse cancers when everything else has failed, reversing heart disease is a piece of cake. And Dr. Dean Ornish has published this extensively in the *Journal of the American Medical Association* as well as the prestigious *Lancet* (*Ornish*). He put folks with arteriosclerosis of important heart (coronary) vessels, on a modified macrobiotic diet. This enabled them to reduce symptoms, reduce medications, and reverse their heart disease by actually shrinking the plaque that had built up in their arteries. Once again God's harmony of His chemistry in the body with His chemistry in foods has brought about healing, when everything that high tech medicine could offer had been exhausted.

For example, scientists found that a component of sesame seeds, an important part of the macrobiotic diet called gomasio (explained in the **Macro Trilogy** - *You Are What You Ate, The Cure Is In the Kitchen* and *Macro Mellow*) has a strong ability to regulate the genes that keep our blood vessels from abnormally producing deadly clots (*Chen*). In fact the phytochemicals in the sesame seeds did a better job if the seeds were whole as opposed to isolating a few of the important components and giving those. Again, this example out of thousands shows that God's biochemical plan in our foods is more potent for healing than anything man can even copy or synthesize. Likewise brown rice, which is an important component of the macrobiotic diet, accelerates the detoxification of cancer-causing chemicals like PCBs (*Sera*). There are literally thousands of references explaining why the macrobiotic diet is so healing even in the face of diseases that medicine is absolutely powerless against.

If you want to learn how to do the diet, start with *You Are What You Ate* first, since this is the primer that shows you how to begin the diet. Next go to the strict healing phase of the complete diet explained in *The Cure Is In the Kitchen*. *Macro Mellow* is a recipe and cookbook that accompanies them (all 3 are available from prestigepublishing.com or 1-800-846-6687 individually or as the *Macro Trilogy*). If you're also interested in the scientific proof of how and why this diet is so effective, read *Tired or Toxic* and past issues of *Total Wellness* (*TW*).

The Not So Sweet Truth
About Sugar Causing Hypertension

Did you ever wonder how we produce rats with high blood pressure for scientific experiments? Do you think we give them a nagging wife or high-pressured job? No. One way researchers can create hypertensive rats is to simply feed them sugar. Like any dietary *faux pas*, sugar causes disease by more than one mechanism. First, most foods containing sugar, like candy, donuts, cookies, pies and cakes also contain damaging trans fatty acids that you learned about in Chapter III. And sugar-containing goodies usually contain bleached flour and lots of chemical names, all of which further indicate the product is highly processed and lacks nutrients necessary for control of blood pressure and sugar, like chromium, manganese, magnesium, and vanadium.

These trace minerals are not only important in preventing hypertension and arteriosclerosis or hardening of the arteries (I'll show you more about nutrients in the next chapter), but they are also necessary for the proper metabolism of sugar itself. And when sugar is not metabolized thoroughly or there is just too much of it for the body to handle, the leftovers in the body literally fry crucial regulatory proteins, damaging their actions, leading to arteriosclerosis or premature aging of blood vessels. This sugar and body protein reaction, called glycosylation, is a major aging mechanism and produces the lipofucsin deposits on the skin that we call "old age spots". And this frying of crucial body proteins by sugar, glycosylation, is a major mechanism contributing to hypertension (*Preuss*).

The solution is not only to eat less sugar, but satisfy your sweet tooth with more nutrient-rich sweets, like fresh, frozen or high antioxidant fruits to restore the missing minerals like chromium, which are lost even faster when you eat sugar. It is another of those vicious cycles where the more sugar you eat, the more chromium you lose. The more chromium you lose, the more sugar you crave. Hence, you are continually eating more sugar and losing more chromium, then craving more, eating more, and gaining more weight, etc. Meanwhile the steady loss of chromium and other nutrients leads to **Syndrome X** with chronic hypertension, escalating weight out of control, fatigue, and the continual birth of multiple new symptoms. Clearly, when you avoid processed foods, you also automatically cut down on sugar as well as trans fatty acids, both potent, yet silent causes of high blood pressure (*Al-Karadaghi*).

The National Cancer Institute has tragically been decades behind what is known in science to successfully prevent and heal cancer (scientific evidence in *TW* 1999-present). When they are recommending you boost their previous five helpings of fruits and vegetables a day to nine as they are now (*Parker-Pope*), you know they realize they have failed you. However, nine servings are not as impossible as they might appear. Most of these "servings" are on average half a cup, which is about the size of a scoop of ice cream or seven cotton balls. Exceptions are for salad greens that are one-cup servings, about the size of your fist or a baseball. And French fries (loaded with trans fatty acids) *do not* count as a vegetable! Never eat them unless homemade with good oil.

Simple things like adding a glass of carrot juice to breakfast can give you another veggie serving. As I have referenced in *TW*, Harvard researchers have shown high doses of beta-carotene transformed (reprogrammed) the p53 cancer gene back to normal. This is one reason why the program which includes frequent carrot juicing in *Wellness Against All Odds* has been proven to more than quadruple cancer survival. Adding a tomato to your salad gives another veggie serving, while having a snack of an apple is another serving. So it's really not difficult to get in all those veggies and fruits if you are focused on better health for yourself and your family. To go even a giant step further, learn how to make whole-grain cold salads that travel well and are delicious, like the barley/walnut/tamari/veggie salad in *Macro Mellow*. For as I will show you, whole grains have even higher antioxidant capacity than do fresh fruits and vegetables.

And don't be hoodwinked by the about-face of McDonald's and other fast food restaurants that are bragging about carrying fast food salads. Their new crispy chicken bacon ranch salad with dressing, for example, has more fat (51 grams) and calories (661) and just as much cholesterol as the Big Mac which has 34 grams of fat and 590 calories (*Leung*). At $4, this heart attack special is not a bargain. Also avoid salads with iceberg lettuce since it has hardly any nutritional value, and likewise avoid salads with canned tuna, which is high in mercury. I prefer to know the source of my foods as much as possible (**Seafood Direct** has a catalog of non-farmed canned fishes).

The irony is that bringing your own food is not only infinitely more healthful, but it's cheaper. So regardless of where you are asked for lunch, if you're not certain of the quality of the food, why not bring your own or suggest a brownbag lunch in fresh air in the park? It's a no-brainer to improved health. If we guard our breakfasts and lunches to make them as health boosting as possible, how bad can dinner be?

Whole Grains Have Twice the Anti-Oxidants

You've been brainwashed to include more fruits and vegetables in your diet because they increase your antioxidant status. But did you know that whole grains are far more important for your antioxidant status than fruits and vegetables? In one study of 88 folks with high blood pressure, 73% of those who had two meals of whole grains a day dropped their blood pressure medication in half in addition to dropping their cholesterol and blood sugar (*Pins*). What are whole grains? Brown rice, millet, quinoa, amaranth, corn, whole wheat, buckwheat, barley, oats, and much more. They are delicious and should be part of your standard cooking. They are described in *Macro Mellow*. And don't forget whole grains increase the cancer fighting ability of the cell as well as decrease the risk of the #3 most common cancer, colon cancer. This should convince you to have the "birdseed cereal" for breakfast and to add a whole grain salad for lunch or dinner (*Macro Mellow* has recipes). What could be an easier start to boosting your vascular health?

Belated as they are, government recommendations for increasing fruits and vegetables have finally been widely promoted. However they've missed the boat by first recommending 5 a day, then 9 which confused folks on how to get that many in, especially since most are overweight. Then only recently has the government finally acknowledged publicly that folks should eat whole grains. But due to food lobbyists' efforts, it is clouded in deceit as far as package labeling goes (*Munoz*), and they failed to really teach the public what whole grains are. Truth be known, you probably cannot get adequate whole grains from any boxed supermarket foods. And I've shown you how to get them, plus they are far less expensive, not genetically damaged and are organic to boot, from **Natural Lifestyle** (1-800-752-2775), my favorite source for non-GMO organic whole grains, beans, seed, nuts, teas, and much more.

Clearly we need more folks aware that whole grains like brown rice, millet, quinoa, buckwheat, barley, oats and other whole grains are an enormous source of anti-oxidants. In fact, **whole grains have more than twice the antioxidant activity of fruits and vegetables.** Folks who have diets containing daily whole grains have 26% less heart disease, 36% fewer strokes, and a 43% lower cancer rate. How simple and inexpensive compared with getting any of these diseases!

You can have grain salads or grain soups for lunch (*Macro Mellow* for recipes), and replace those trans fatty acid-laden French fries with brown rice and other whole grains at dinner, for starters.

Serial Killers in Your Pantry?

If you have boxed breakfast cereals in your pantry, two to one they are silently eroding your health. Think about it. One of the most important meals of the day is relegated to companies that load cereals with hydrogenated oils that contain damaging trans fatty acids. As I highly referenced in *Detoxify or Die*, these have been shown by Harvard researchers to clearly promote the epidemic of high cholesterol, which is now seen merely as a deficiency of coenzyme Q10-depleting statin drugs. Boxed breakfast cereals also contain sugars that rob you of minerals, plus additives and dyes that needlessly overwork your detoxification system. Whenever a food is "fortified" that should be a clear warning that so much has been removed through the work of processing that the addition of a handful of cheap synthetic nutrients is mandated. After all, nature doesn't need to be fortified.

As well, boxed grocery store cereals often contain bleached and pulverized grains that have been dead for months and stripped of their vitamin E. In fact when serious modern day trans-Atlantic sailors begin a long trip, they often put their cereals in plastic bags for the voyage to stop little bugs from being attracted on board. What are the bugs attracted to? Not the actual cereal, but the box it comes in. Pretty ironic that they find more nutrition in the packaging!

Studies now conclusively show that **natural vitamin E cuts the heart attack and cancer rates by more than one-third**. In addition if you have cancer, it makes cancer cells even more sensitive to killing by radiation, while at the same time it makes normal body cells resistant to radiation damage and decreases the side effects from these carcinogenic treatments. Therefore it is inconceivable that there would be any oncologists or radiation therapists recommending radiation therapy for cancers who do not prescribe natural vitamin E and foods containing it. Although beyond the scope of this book, I've given lots more cancer fighting plans in back issues of *TW*, especially 1999-2005, complete with evidence.

Like a serial killer, these boxed cereals, which make up one-third of many Americans' diets, stealthily help create disease and death. Dr. Lorraine Day, former chief orthopedic surgeon at San Francisco General Hospital, years ago developed breast cancer. She graciously gave me photographs and laboratory reports so that I could show slides of these when I was lecturing to physicians at Oxford University. In the lecture ("The scientific basis for reversing end-stage cancer") I showed how her breast cancer went from grape size to grapefruit size in one month and how 2 major medical centers had confirmed the biopsy reports as metastatic infiltrating ductal adenocarcinoma. Yet this surgeon did not have surgery and did not have chemotherapy. Instead she ate a live or raw whole foods diet plus many of the things that you can read about in *Wellness Against All Odds*, a natural non-prescription program proven to more than quadruple cancer survival (references in *TW* 2000, and Dr. Day's excellent videos are available at 1-800-574-2437).

Just what is a live or raw food diet? Eating as much as you can in the raw, natural state, which amounts to about 85%. Any grains, nuts, seeds or beans are soaked or sprouted to improve taste and digestibility. Why uncooked food? Because food that has not been cooked (or mutilated in a factory) has more nutrition, while heat, processing, and time destroy nutrients. In addition, there are live enzymes in recently live food that can be used by the body for a variety of purposes, like detoxification of the colon and bloodstream, improving digestion, improving lymphatic flow and more. And past *TW* issues show the medical evidence that enzymes help break down the protective armor around bacteria (biofilms) and cancers (sialoglycoproteins), making them much easier targets for the immune system. So if whole foods are so good for a tough disease like cancer, think what they can do for your blood vessel health.

Birdseed Cereal

Now let's take another look at that birdseed cereal, for I want to make it incredibly easy for you. Before bed merely put equal parts of raw (not roasted) buckwheat groats and raw (not roasted or salted) sunflower seeds (usually ¼ cup of each) and a small handful of raw almonds in a bowl. Just add water before you go to bed, and drain it in the morning. Then the fun begins; add blueberries, pineapple, chopped dates, or whatever your heart desires or nothing. You can add fruit juices, dried or fresh fruits, yogurt (the one with the cream on top---yum), kefir, nut milks, grain milks like amasake (a sweet rice milk), sweeteners like maple syrup, molasses, honey, or yinnie rice syrup.

Voila! You have live raw grains and seeds so full of nutrition that they could start a whole plant. In fact, I usually soak enough for three days at a time, so by the third day some are starting to sprout little roots and leaves. The variety is endless as you can use any grains, seeds, and nuts that you desire as well as any fruits (dried or fresh), juice (fruit, nut or grain milks, yogurt) and optional sweetener (maple syrup, dates, honey, etc). For travel, merely mix your "birdseed cereal" in a baggie or jar and bring along a bowl and a spoon and a couple of fruits (or dried fruits). Soak the amount you want to eat for breakfast overnight and add cut up fruits to it the next morning. You have an inexpensive, portable, highly nutritious breakfast with live whole grains bursting with nutrition versus dead hotel "food".

Don't forget buckwheat is not a member of the wheat family, which our diets are so overloaded with. Wheat can trigger opioid receptors in the brain, leading to addiction to it, and the gluten in wheat can cause serious intestinal damage at any time in life leading to malabsorption of nutrients, as well as depression and arthritis (more on that in *Wellness Against All Odds*). In addition as we showed in October 2003 *TW*, gluten-triggered celiac disease can masquerade as any symptom, begin at any time, and is insidiously on the rise with very few physicians diagnosing it. Buckwheat (not a member of the wheat family) is also beneficial in improving cholesterol levels as well as blood sugar in diabetics.

Within a few days of the "birdseed breakfast" painful hemorrhoids can shrink down, constipation disappears, then blood toxicity clears. But always remember that nothing is for everyone. Folks with colitis often find raw foods intolerable and need to heal the gut first. *No More Heartburn* provides you with all of the details for healing the gut.

It's pretty sad when the majority of the country is spending more money than they need to on a breakfast that is robbing them of health. The "birdseed breakfast" is infinitely less expensive and does not contain trans fatty acids that slowly accumulate and damage cell membranes, leading to every disease including cancer. As well, it avoids the many additives, dyes, pesticides, sugars, chemical names, genetically modified oils and other junk that is in commercial boxed cereals. This should convince you to have the "birdseed cereal" for breakfast and a whole grain salad for lunch or dinner (*Macro Mellow* contains the recipes). What could be easier? Empower yourself to new heights. It's time to make sure your breakfast cereal is not a serial killer.

Forget Those Unpalatable Low Salt Diets

One of the first dietary recommendations given to folks with hypertension is for a low salt diet. But this torture that makes everything taste like cardboard often fails. Why? Because once again they are working blindly and without the answers to all your wonderful chemistry at their fingertips. Sure, cutting down on salt should lower the water-holding ability of your vessels, and like any plumbing situation, that lowers the pressure. But they forgot to ask why your natural salt regulation is on the fritz, and how they might permanently fix it without torturing you.

It turns out that salt's sodium is controlled by a membrane enzyme system ($Na+K+-ATPase$) that is controlled in part by your oil change that you learned about in Chapter III.

And the other part of salt control is via magnesium (Chapter I) and vitamin C (Chapter II) (*Skou, Farvid*). Correct them all, and you usually (barring any other concomitant deficiencies or a kidney toxic with cadmium or lead, Chapter IV) no longer have salt-induced hypertension.

Capitalize With Your Most Powerful Vegetable

I know that you know you should eat your vegetables, but in case you are caught short, do you know the most important ones that you want at least once and preferably twice a day? Brassica or cruciferous vegetables, which include cabbage, broccoli, cauliflower, Brussels sprouts, kale, collard greens, watercress, turnips, radishes, mustard greens, horseradish, mizuna, cilantro, and more. I showed you in *Detoxify or Die* how they protect from breast and other cancers, but they go far beyond that (*Chiao*).

Cruciferous veggies rev up both phases of detoxification plus glutathione production (*Maheo, Kassahun, Ye*). That means they are protecting you in a variety of ways every day against the onslaught of environmental chemicals that are propelling you not only toward high blood pressure, but cancer and every other malady. In fact in one study, two half-cup servings of Brassica a day rev up your detoxification of drugs like Tylenol nearly 20%. What drug can do that?

So how do you make sure you get these? Cabbage salad at lunch is easy (without trans fatty acid mayo—make your own via *Macro Mellow*). Then add any of the others at dinner. I even like to sneak a small portion of kale onto Luscious' Sunday plate of scrambled eggs with salmon and onion slice on trans fatty acid-free organic bread or croissant. Cauliflower can be mashed and seasoned to resemble mashed potatoes, broccoli makes delicious soup, and don't neglect a small salad of watercress, mizuna and/or arugula for lunch, dinner or brunch! Use your wonderfully creative imagination. And if you still can't get them in? **IndolPlex** two twice a day will do the trick.

The most impressive medical studies on the powerful detoxification-boosting Brassica were actually done on broccoli sprouts. You can get **organic non-GMO broccoli seeds** and make your own delicious broccoli sprouts for salads, soups, sandwiches and garnishes from Natural Lifestyle (natural-lifestyle.com, 1-800-752-2775)

Healthful Chocolate That Heals Vessels?

Do you think that everything that is good for you is on the bad list? Well, guess again. It turns out that dark chocolate derived from the cacao bean plant is a rich source of flavonoids. Flavonoids are strong antioxidants and protect the heart, inhibit clots, and stimulate nitric oxide inside the blood vessel, the gas you learned about that turns off abnormal clots plus relaxes and dilates our blood vessels (*Engler*). Dark chocolate high in flavonoids, procyanidins and epicatechins is so beneficial that smart manufacturers should start putting these concentrations on their wrappers. But look for **very dark rich chocolate, not milk chocolate,** and chocolate that does not contain any hydrogenated, partially hydrogenated, polyunsaturated or vegetable oils or shortening (no trans fatty acids!). The European dark chocolate bars with lecithin, absolutely no artificial flavorings and no artificial colorings nor trans fatty acid laden-fats or oils are usually the real thing. Make sure you understand what every ingredient is. Meanwhile, give yourself and your sweetie chocolate, but make sure it's good and dark.

Healing With Water

We know clean water is a nearly an extinct entity when it costs over six times more than gasoline. Currently bottled water goes for anywhere from $8-$16 per gallon whereas gasoline is hovering over $2 a gallon. You've read in *DOD* about the epidemics of childhood leukemia from industrial TCE (trichloroethylene) in city water supplies. Then you saw in *TW* the reports from the *USA Today* cover article showing that over half the United States cities have levels of TCE that are beyond safe limits. Meanwhile, Texas newspapers report that the fish caught in lakes have measurable levels of Prozac in them. Why? Because the millions of people on this drug urinate out Prozac which then goes into the wastewater treatment plants. But we have no chemicals to degrade Prozac, antibiotics, chemotherapy drugs (which can also cause cancer), hormones, and many other drugs. So these drugs go right into the streams and rivers unchanged and are taken up by the fish (and us).

Clearly everyone knows they need clean water and a filtration system. But most don't know they also need alkaline water. Unfortunately, the majority of waters from the tap and bottled waters are just the opposite, highly acidic. You can get pH paper to test them yourself (from prlabs.com). Most of them test out at about 5.1 on the pH scale. Real water is neutral at 7.0. When our bodies are busy detoxifying the many chemicals we are exposed to all day in our air, food, and water it makes the body acidic. And when we eat an acid diet of sweets, sodas, sugars, processed foods or a lot of meat, the body gets even more acidic. Likewise when the body is fighting off infection, is burdened with damaging emotions or with a chronic disease like diabetes, or is trying to heal, it also is acidic. And when Mr. ED (endothelial dysfunction) rears his head, you are acidic. In fact when someone shows up in the emergency room with near death coma, one of the treatments is to alkalinize or neutralize this acidity to reverse it. Therefore it makes sense that we should be drinking alkaline water to help the body save its buffering or neutralizing calcium and other minerals for better uses, like preventing osteoporosis or high blood pressure.

Alkalinize or Deteriorate

Acidity can be subtle. When the body is overly acidic it causes a deep sighing respiration and frequent yawning. Acidity hampers the heart strength and energy and it slows the metabolism in the body in general and leads to hypoglycemia (low blood sugar with sudden headaches, sweating, irritability, rage, faintness, dizziness and more). Also when the body is acidic it shifts the oxygen dissociation curve of hemoglobin to the right. To non-physicians this means it makes it harder for the body to get oxygen out of the red blood cells and into the blood vessel lining (endothelial cells) and other tissues where it is needed for the chemistry of life.

The effect of acidosis on the nervous system can range from mood swings, fatigue and abnormal drowsiness to coma. Acidity affects the kidneys as well, making them produce more ammonia to try to neutralize or offset the acidity. This in turn wastes proteins and can lead to hypertension by another mechanism. Furthermore, a body on the acid side uses up a lot of calcium to offset or neutralize the acidity. When the body runs out of its buffering calcium it steals it from the bone, leading to osteopenia and osteoporosis. And worst of all, when our bodies are too acidic, this hampers the normal metabolism of the cell making it more difficult for it to clean out and eliminate daily toxicity. Thus the cell builds up in toxic wastes and this accelerates aging and robs us of energy.

On the flip side, the advantages of alkaline water are clear:
- It improves the strength of the heart by making calcium and glucose more available,
- it improves circulation by making it easier for oxygen to get out of the red blood cell and into the body tissues for nurturing and healing,
- it improves the metabolism, energy and detoxification of all cells, and
- it puts a damper on the loss of minerals that would be used as buffers, like calcium, from bone, thus slowing down osteoporosis (*Ledingham, Plaskett, Groff*).

That's why the **Alkaline Water Machine** (a.k.a. the Spring Ionizer) is so important an appliance in your kitchen. It easily attaches to your faucet so that you can merely flick the lever whenever you want to make healthful alkaline water (hightechhealth.com or 1-800-794-5355). If you haven't already added this to your kitchen, isn't it about time you did?

Alkalinize or Die

Clearly as the body becomes sicker, it becomes more acidic. Think of diabetic acidosis that can lead to coma and death. Without insulin, the body cannot move glucose into the cell for energy creation, leaving unbuffered acids to build up that can bring life to a screeching halt. Overwhelming infection also creates an acidity in the body, as does trauma as from an accident, for example. And even well honed athletes when they push their bodies too far can develop acidosis, as lactic acid builds up in muscles causing exhaustion and cramping. Unfortunately regular tap water and the majority of bottled waters do not help this problem at all, because they are highly acidic, usually with a pH of around 5.1. The body prefers a pH of around 7.34 in the alkaline range for maximum performance.

And folks who drink fizzy or carbonated drinks are even in more danger, because the carbon dioxide forms carbonic acid, which makes the water even more acidic and pulls out more calcium. This makes the body more vulnerable for any disease, since it makes the body's buffering system work overtime trying to neutralize excess acidity. Diets high in sugars and processed foods lead to further acidity, depleting buffering (which now makes the body steal calcium from the bones as an emergency buffer), fostering osteoporosis, hypertension, and many more diseases.

Furthermore, cholesterol is only damaging and only plasters itself on blood vessel walls when it is oxidized by free radicals. Otherwise, unoxidized cholesterol is not only harmless, but also necessary for multiple biochemical steps in the process of life. But free radicals change cholesterol so that it can now get a death-grip on the vessel wall and start stiffening arterial walls or plugging them up. These free radicals that come from metabolizing the chemicals in our air, food, and water are naked electrons that wildly steal electrons from cholesterol molecules. This results in oxidized cholesterol molecules, which now are missing their own electrons. So they in turn wildly attack the endothelial lining of the blood vessel. They are merely looking for an electron as another mate. But by grabbing onto the blood vessel wall to snatch that electron, it glues the cholesterol plaque to the artery. This eventually grows and plugs off the artery and leads to hardening, calcification, hypertension, stroke, ruptured aneurysms or heart attack. High doses of antioxidants are part of the cure to slow this damage by sopping up these free radicals like a sponge before they oxidize cholesterol.

Besides free radicals in our blood burning holes in the lining of blood vessel walls, also bacteria like H. pylori do, as you learned in Chapter III. This makes the body send out an urgent call for its cholesterol Band-Aid to patch up the holes before we bleed to death. Hence, we have another free radical-mediated mechanism for triggering high blood pressure, high cholesterol or heart attacks. Once more the amount of antioxidant protection we have makes the difference between early aging, early disease or none.

Wouldn't it be wonderful if we had something simple that could alkalinize (buffer or neutralize) free radicals in the body before they cause their destruction? And wouldn't it be even more wonderful if this also served as a free radical sponge, sopping up disease-producing free radicals as they wander about the body? We can rescue the body from this disease-producing acidity and excess free radicals by putting it in the alkaline zone. We can accomplish both feats with one healthful remedy that has even additional benefits.

In *Detoxify or Die*, I showed you on page 22 how the **Alkaline Water Machine** (High Tech Health 1-800-794-5355) is superior to reverse osmosis machines for removing unwanted chemicals from tap water. As well, through a patented electrolysis of water, the Alkaline Water Machine can provide any degree of alkalinization of your drinking water that you want with the push of a button. But it does more.

Alkaline Water as an Antioxidant and Bone-Sparing Buffer

If that were not enough of a reason for using this machine for your primary water source, it also has superior antioxidant ability. Active hydrogen is produced near the cathode during the electrolysis or alkalinization of the water. At the cathode, the hydrogen ion gains electrons, changing it into active hydrogen that has a high reducing potential, meaning it is a very powerful free radical sponge. This results in an alkaline or high pH with high dissolved hydrogen, which scavenges free radicals. It is such a good free radical sponge that it **performs as well as the primary antioxidant enzymes that the body makes, namely superoxide dismutase (SOD) and catalase. And it even does a better job than SOD,** because SOD produces hydrogen peroxide that then has to be neutralized. Hydrogen peroxide (H_2O_2) is one free radical that turns on cancer metastases. But reduced water does not produce this unwanted free radical. As well, reduced or alkalinized water suppresses genetic DNA breakage or mutation while it scavenges over four types of free radicals (*Shirahata*).

Since alkalinize water can prevent DNA damage by peroxide, hydroxyl, and oxy radicals, it should have an important role not only for everyday use, but especially in defending us against all types of degenerative diseases, including not only high blood pressure, but cancers. The main mechanism of metastases of cancers is through free radical damage. So for all-around health it certainly makes the best sense to choose the **Alkaline Water Machine** for purifying, alkalinizing, free radical-fighting, gene-protecting, cholesterol-suppressing, water. It attaches simply to any water faucet. Where else can you get 4 functions rolled into the most healthful water possible? You may have never given water much thought, but alkaline water is definitely one of your weapons against high blood pressure.

Green Tea Lowers High Blood Pressure

Green tea contains polyphenols, God-given chemicals that include such difficult chemical names as epigallocatechin-3 gallate (EGCG). These wouldn't be worth learning about if they didn't have strong anticancer effects. And since they are natural antioxidants, you guessed it, they also decrease death from heart attacks (*Hertzog, Kono*) and reduce arteriosclerosis as well as cholesterol deposits in blood vessels (*Vinson*). Green tea polyphenols dramatically reduced the incidence of cardiovascular disease in many more studies (*Seno,Chyu*). As well, they have reduced blood pressure (*Negishi*). With a myriad of benefits, it makes incredible sense to be sipping on green tea throughout the day rather than coffee or sodas. If you prefer high quality non-GMO organic foods as I do, you can get your teas from the **Natural Lifestyle** catalog.

With everyone walking and driving around these days clutching a soda, it makes sense to substitute these high fructose GMO corn-syrup sodas for healthful green tea. For not only is over 40% of the corn from which these sugars are derived from genetically engineered corn, but also the fructose contributes to arteriosclerosis (*Benado*). Take tea and see how you feel.

Garlic to the Rescue

You can imagine my surprise as a physician for over a quarter of a century to learn that this ancient herb not only lowers blood pressure, but makes the blood clotting cells or platelets, less able to clump together to form fatal clots. And it lowers cholesterol (*Harenberg, Neil, McMahon, Santo, Rietz, Orekhov, Wagner, Durak*). Garlic lowers blood pressure, in part, because it acts like an ACE inhibitor, but without the nasty side effects or cost of this commonly prescribed anti-hypertensive drug category. Garlic can also trigger the vasodilating gas, NO (nitric oxide) by yet another mechanism to lower blood pressure (*Das*). Wow! Mother Nature is amazing, for no drug does all that, and if it did, it sure would not be able to do it without side effects as garlic can.

Keep Your Arteries Clean With Kyolic

In one study, they purposely fed a high cholesterol diet to rabbits. As predicted, they developed dense arteriosclerotic plaque in the body's main artery, the aorta. But in another group that was fed garlic extract, there was significant reduction in the amount of plaque. In fact the photographs of their aortas looked just like the clean ones of the control group that was not fed a high cholesterol diet (*Durak*).

There is only one garlic on the market that has over 300 research studies behind its biochemistry and human effects. Kyolic is aged by a proprietary process that fosters more antioxidant effects than other types. Use one teaspoon of

Kyolic Liquid (equivalent to 4 capsules) four times a day for lowering cholesterol, improving antioxidant capability, lowering homocysteine (the only form of garlic proven to do this), thwarting cancers, limiting platelet stickiness (making them less likely to clot), and much more.

With over two decades of volumes of research, I can't help but wonder what other benefits Kyolic must have when it has so many. I've included lots of key references here because I know it seems too good to be true for anyone who is not familiar with all the science behind garlic (*Wagner, Rietz, Lau, Pennsylvania State University and the National Cancer Institute, Makheja, Bordia, Harenberg, Neil, McMahon, Santo, Orekhov, Das*). Kyolic (made by Wakunaga) is a special form of aged garlic to mature the factors that have the most potency and cardio-protection. Why not get some free samples of Kyolic, just by mentioning this book (1-800-825-7888)? Then take 2 twice a day to lower your pressure. The form I like best is the powerful **Kyolic Liquid** because one tsp is equivalent to 4 capsules, and it's easy to slip the bottle into your pocket and just give a big squirt down your throat 3-5 times a day. Don't worry, there is no garlic odor. Isn't it amazing how simple the relief for hypertension can be for some folks? For remember, *garlic is a potent activator of nitric oxide synthase (Das)*, the enzyme the body uses to make vasodilating NO (nitric oxide). Hypertension is not a deficiency of drugs (that can give you even higher blood pressure), in fact the drugs put you on a fast track for accelerated aging. Food is a major factor in healing, yet our food sources have been so compromised by processing that they clearly foster degeneration and disease. Now you have numerous tools with which to counter this for yourself and family.

The Seaweed Solution

There is a healthful component of the cancer-reversing macrobiotic diet that you could easily incorporate into your
daily anti-aging vascular protection diet. That's seaweed!
Sea vegetables are loaded with minerals and fatty acids of
the omega-3 type. In fact, fish that are your major source of
vessel-healing omega-3 cod liver oil get theirs from sea
vegetables. There are many varieties of sea vegetables and
you can sneak them into soups and a host of other delicious
dishes. Wakame contains substances that mimic the commonly prescribed anti-hypertensive drugs, called the angiotensin-converting enzyme inhibitors (or ACE inhibitors), but
without their nasty side effects. And as the usual bonus that
you get in beneficial side effects with foods, you get trace
minerals (*Suetsuna, Nakano, Li*).

You may recall from Chapter I that some of the 27 medications that are ACE (or angiotensin converting enzyme) inhibitors include such names as Accupril, Altace, Captopril,
Lotensin, Monopril, Prinivil, Univasc, Vasotec, Zestril, Accuretic (an ACE inhibitor with a diuretic, hydrochlorothiazide),
Aceon, Atacand, Avalide (this ACE inhibitor also contains a
diuretic), Avapro, Capoten, Capozide (also with a diuretic),
Cozaar, Diovan, and more. A veritable alphabet soup! They,
like all drugs, have pages of side effects in the book of drugs,
PDR (*Physician's Desk Reference*). Why not learn how to slide
Nature's gift of sea vegetables into your meals? Two short
recipe books to get you started are *Sea Vegetable Celebration*
(seaveg.com or fax: 207-565-2144) and *Macro Mellow* (presti-
gepublishing.com or 1-800-846-6687).

How else can you ease your family into the idea of eating sea vegetables? When it gets pretty hectic around your house, you know there are going to be missed meals, and that you'll find candy bar wrappers as evidence of what really was eaten. As Marie Antoinette might have said, so then let them eat candy. But that doesn't mean they have to eat junk. The company that harvests sea vegetables for macrobiotic and other diets, Maine Coast Sea Vegetables, Inc., makes healthful candy bars.

Kelp Crunch, also called **Maine Coast Crunch,** comes in two crunchy chewy flavors, soy nut ginger and original sesame (seaveg.com). The great news is they are 100% organic and GMO-free, and are whole foods energy bars of sesame seeds, soy nuts, kelp, brown rice syrup, maple syrup and (optional) ginger. One bar has over 74 mg of magnesium and 155 mg of calcium plus 20 mcg of folic acid. Just those ingredients alone would be hard to beat by other bars. And no worry about junk. There is none.

Healthful Chips? No Longer an Oxymoron

Everywhere you go chips and dips are universal foods for entertaining. It always amazes me at events hosted by people with more money than they know what to do with to see them actually putting chips in their bodies. Then they wonder why they spend so much time and money on doctor visits and drugs, and don't feel vivaciously well. Clearly you have to have your head examined to eat chips, because they are loaded with disease-producing trans fatty acids, a major cause of high cholesterol, high LDL, high triglycerides and low "good" HDL cholesterol. Not only that, they damage all cell membrane chemistry so that high blood pressure, allergies, heart disease, Alzheimer's and more are triggered. If that weren't enough, potato chips are a great source of night-shades which trigger arthritis of all sorts, tendonitis, back pain blamed on deteriorating disks, and much more (see *Pain Free in 6 Weeks* for details, prestigepublishing.com).

As a result, I haven't had a chip in a couple of decades. In fact you couldn't pay me to eat them since my paralyzed leg for two months from an inadvertent ingestion of nightshades. Likewise even chips that are made out of corn contain "spices" which invariably include the hidden night-shades paprika, cayenne or chili. As well, chips usually contain trans fatty acids anyway. So you'll be pleased to learn about healthful chips made out of organic corn and sea vegetables with no trans fatty acids and no nightshades!

Maine Coast Sea Vegetables, Inc., famous in macrobiotic circles for decades for top-quality sea vegetables (and the healthful candy bars you just learned about), makes chips with 100% organic ingredients which include organic corn, organic safflower or sunflower oil, organic sea vegetables, dulse and kelp, plus organic onion and garlic. And the bottom line is they are healthful, delicious and not loaded with salt, so you do not wake up with high blood pressure, puffy eyes, swollen ankles, or bloated in the morning.

As you just learned, sea vegetables, are used to control blood pressure as well as prescription drugs do, but without their long list of side effects. (*Suetsuna*). In addition, sea vegetables provide you with healthful minerals and fatty acids that the blood pressure drugs sure don't. And remember all the hype about making sure you eat fish a couple of times a week to get good omega-3 oils in your system to prevent cancers, heart attacks and other illnesses? Unknowledgeable sources who recommend eating more fish are oblivious to the fact that most of it is farm raised and raises your deadly mercury levels. Farmed fish also have about 10 times the cancer-causing PCBs of wild fish. But where do you think fish get their wonderful omega-3 levels? From eating God's sea vegetables.

Just ask your local health food store or grocery store to carry **Sea Chips** by Maine Coast Sea Vegetables, Inc., in Franklin Maine, or go to their Web site seaveg.com or call 207-565-2907. You can also get Sea Chips and the healthful **Kelp Crunch** energy bars from Natural Lifestyle, the catalog source for your organic, non-GMO grains, beans, seeds, nuts, and more. Then use your *Macro Mellow* cookbook (prestigepublishing.com or 1-800-846-6687) to make delicious humus and other healthful bean and vegetable dips for your delightful **Sea Chips**. In fact next time you are invited to a cocktail party, offer to bring the chips and dips, and then you'll know that there'll be something healthful that you can eat and enjoy. Let the rest of them eat the other junk chips laden with arthritis-producing nightshades and disease-accelerating trans fatty acids, while you dine on health-promoting **Sea Chips**!

Product Sources:

- Alkaline Water Machine, High Tech Health, 1-800-794-5355
- Complexed Potassium, Carlson, 1-800-323-4141
- Kyolic, Wakunaga, 1-800-421-2998
- Kyo-Green, Wakunaga, 1-800-421-2998
- Organic grains, beans, nuts, teas, Natural Lifestyle, 1-800-752-2775
- Broccoli seeds for sprouting, Natural Lifestyle, 1-800-752-2775
- Kelp Crunch, Sea Chips, Natural Lifestyle, 1-800-752-2775
- Safer seafood, Seafood Direct, 1-800-732-1836
- Maine Coast Sea Vegetables for cooking, recipe book, plus Kelp Crunch, Sea Chips, seaveg.com, 207-565-2907, fax: 207-565-2144
- IndolPlex (Integrative Therapeutics) NEEDS, 1-800-634-1380

References:

Le OT, Elliott WJ, Dose response relationship of blood pressure and serum cholesterol to 3-N-butyl phthalide, a component of celery oil, *Clin Res*, 39:750 A, 1991

Maizes V, Integrative approaches to hypertension, *Clinics Fam Practice*, 4; 4:895-905, 2002

Le OT, Elliot WJ, Mechanisms of the hypotensive effect of 3-N-butyl phthalide (BUPH): a component of celery oil. *J Am Hypertens* 40:326 A, 1992

Rogers SA, *Detoxify or Die*, 2002, prestigepublishing.com or 1-800-846-6687

Rogers SA, *No More Heartburn*, 2001, prestigepublishing.com or 1-800-846-6687

Rogers SA, *Wellness Against All Odds*, 1994, prestigepublishing.com or 1-800-846-6687

Rogers SA, Gallinger S, *Macro Mellow*, 1992, prestigepublishing.com or 1-800-846-6687

Jones JM, Reicks M, Marquart L, et al, The importance of promoting a whole grain foods message, *J Am Coll Nutr*. 21; 4:293-297, 2002

Kumar B, Jha MN, Prasad KN, et al, D-alpha tocopheryl succinate (vitamin E) enhances radiation-induced chromosomal damage levels in human cancer cells, but reduces it in normal cells. *J Am Coll Nutr*. 21; 4: 339-343, 2002

Ahmud N, Feyes DK, Nieminen AL, et al, Green tea constituent epigallacatechin-3-gallate and induction of apoptosis and cell cycle arrest human carcinoma cells, *J Natl Cancer Inst*; 89:1881-6, 1997

Erba D, Riso P, Colombo A, Testolin G, Supplementation of Jurkat T cells with green tea extract decreases oxidative damage due to iron treatment, *J Nutr*, 129:2130-4, 1999

Katiyar SK, Mmukhtar H, Tea antioxidants in cancer chemoprevention, *J Cell Biochem*; 27:S59-67, 1997

Lee IP, Kim YH, Kang MH, et al, Chemopreventative effect of green tea (*Camellia sinensis*) against cigarette smoke-induced mutations (SCE) in humans, *J Cell Biochem* 1997; 27:S68-75, 1997

Sato D, Inhibition of urinary bladder tumors induced by N-butyl-N-(4-hydroxybutyl)-nitrosamine in rats by green tea, *Int J Urol*, 6:93-99, 1999

Cummins R, Lilliston B, *Genetically engineered food*, Marlowe & Co., New York, 2000 (available 1-800-752-2775)

Ghosh MK Chattopadhyay DJ, Chatterjee IB, Vitamin C prevents oxidative damage, *Free Rad Res* 25: 2: 173-79, 1996

Fine AM, Oligomeric proanthocyanidin complexes: history, structure, and phytopharmaceutical applications, *Altern Med Rev* 5; 2:144-51, 2000

Street JC, Chadwick RW, Ascorbic acid requirements and metabolism in relation to organochlorine pesticides, *Ann NY Acad Sci* 258: 132-43, Sept. 1975

Milner JA, Rivlin RS, Recent advances on the nutritional effects associated with the use of garlic as a supplement, *Journal of Nutrition*, 131; 35, March 2001, ISSN 0022-3166 (This whole issue was devoted to Kyolic and its molecular biochemistry with dozens of papers by outstanding scientists from medical schools throughout the United States and the world, detailing its cholesterol-lowering, antioxidant, detoxification boosting, cancer inhibiting, antihypertensive, antibiotic-like, and many other properties: physicians can get a copy from Wakunaga.)

Kasuga S, et al, Pharmacologic activities of aged garlic extract in comparison with other garlic preparations, 1080, ibid, Milner.

Numagami Y, S-allylcysteine inhibits free radical production, lipid peroxidation and neuronal damage in rat brain ischemia, 1100, ibid, Milner.

Sivam G, Protection against *Helicobacter pylori* and other bacterial infections by garlic, 1106, ibid, Milner.

Hoshino T, Effects of garlic preparations on the gastrointestinal mucosal, 1109, ibid, Milner.

Lamm DL, Riggs TR, Enhanced immunocompetence by garlic role in bladder cancer and other malignancies, 1067 s, ibid, Milner

Scheer JF, Allison L, Fox C, *The Garlic Cure*, 2002, Alpha-Omega Press 3303 Fiechtner Drive, Fargo ND 58103 (1-800-421-2998 ext. 158)

Geng Z, Lau BHS, Aged garlic extract modulates glutathione redox cycle and superoxide dismutase activity in the vascular endothelial cells, *Phytotherapy Research* 11: 54-56

Sumioka I, et al, Mechanisms of protection by S-allylmercaptocysteine against acetaminophen-induced liver injury in mice, *Jpn J Pharmacol* 78: 199-207, 1998

Wakunaga, *Aged Garlic Extract. Research Excerpts from Peer Reviewed Scientific Journals and Scientific Meetings*, Wakunaga, Mission Viejo CA, 1-800-4 21-2998, March 2000

Silagy CA, Neil HA, A meta-analysis of the effect of garlic on blood pressure, *J Hypertens*, 12; 4:463-8, Apr 12, 1994

Joshipura KJ, Ascherio A, Willett WC, et al, Fruit and vegetable intake in relation to risk of ischemic stroke, *J Amer Med Assoc* 282:1233-39, 1999

Gillman MW, Cupples LA, Gagnon D, et al, Protective effect of fruits and vegetables on development of stroke in men, *J Amer Med Assoc* 273:1113-17, 1995.

Plotnick GD, Corretti MC, Vogel RA, Effect of antioxidant vitamins on the transient impairment of endothelium-dependent brachial artery vasoactivity following a single high-fat meal, *J Amer Med Assoc* 278; 20:1682-86, Nov 26, 1997

Ornish D, Scherwitz LW, Brand RJ, et al. Intensive lifestyle changes for reversal of coronary heart disease, *J Am Med Assoc*, 2: 2001-2007, 1998

Ornish DM, Brown SE, Scherwitz LW, et al. Can lifestyle changes reverse coronary heart disease? *Lancet* 336: 129-133, 1990

Preuss HG, Effects of chromium and guar on sugar-induced hypertension in rats, *Clin Nephrology*, 44; 3:170-77, 1995

Preuss HG, Blood pressure response to sucrose ingestion in four strains of rats, *Amer J Hypert* 5:244-50, 1992

Al-Karadaghi P, et al, Renal function and sugar-induced blood pressure elevations, *J Amer Coll Nutr*, 10; 5:556-70, Oct 1991

Negishi H, Xu JW, Yamori Y, et al, Black and green tea polyphenols attenuate blood pressure increases in stroke-prone spontaneously hypertensive rats, *J Nutr*, 134; 1:38-42, Jan. 2004

Kono S, Shinchi K, Imanishi K et al, Green tea consumption and serum lipid profiles: a cross-sectional study in northern Kyushu, Japan, *Prev Med*, 21; 4: 526-31, Jul. 1992

Vinson JA, Teufel K, Wu N, Green and black teas inhibit arteriosclerosis by lipid, antioxidant, and fibrinolytic mechanisms, *J Agricul Food Chem*, 52; 11: 3661-65, Jun. 2, 2004

Sano J, Inami S, Seimiya K, et al, Effects of green tea intake on the development of coronary artery disease, *Circul J*, 68; 7: 665-70, July 2004

177

Chyu KY, Babbidge SM, Zhao X, et al, Differential effects of green tea-derived catechin on developing vs. established arteriosclerosis in apolipoprotein E-null mice, *Circulation*, 109; 20: 2448-53, May 25, 2004

Pins JJ, et al, Do whole-grain oat cereals reduce the need for antihypertensive medications and improve blood pressure control? *J Fam Pract* 51: 353-359, 2002

Ledingham JGG, Warrell DA, *Concise Oxford Textbook of Medicine*, Oxford: Oxford University Press, 2000

Plaskett LG, On the essentiality of dietary carbohydrate, *J Nutr Environ Med* 13; 3:161-68, Sept 2003

Groff JL, Gropper SS, Hunt SM, *Advanced Nutrition and Human Metabolism*, P. 138, West Publishing, 1995

Plaskett LG, *The Wherewithal to Detoxify*, Tiverton: Nutrigold, 2001

Shirahata S, Kabayama S, Nakano M, Katakura Y, et al, Electrolized-reduced water scavenges active oxygen species and protects DNA from oxidative damage, *Biochem Biophys Res Commun*, 234:269-274, 1997

Durak I, Ozturk HS, Olcay E, Guven C, Effects of garlic extract supplementation on blood lipid and antioxidant parameters and atherosclerotic plaque formation process in cholesterol-fed rabbits. *J Herb Pharmacother* 2; 2: 19-32, 2002

Wagner H, et al, Evaluation of natural products as inhibitors of angiotensin 1-converting enzyme (ACE), *Pharm Phamacol Lett* 1:15-18, 1991(garlic as ACE inhibitor)

Rietz B, et al, Cardioprotective actions of wild garlic (Allium ursinum) in ischemia and reperfusion, *Mol Cell Biochem* 119:143-50, 1993

Lau B, *Garlic And You: The Modern Medicine*, Apple Publishing, 220 East 59th Ave, Vancouver BC, Can V5X 1X9, 1997

Pennsylvania State University and the National Cancer Institute, *Aged Garlic Extract, current Research Papers form Peer Reviewed Scientific Journals & Meetings*, Wakunaga, Mission, Viejo CA, (800-421-2998), 1998

Makheja AN, et al, Inhibition of platelet aggregation and thromboxane synthesis by onion and garlic, *Lancet*, 1:781-2, 1979

Bordia T, et al, An evaluation of garlic and onion as antithrombotic agents, *Prostaglandins, Leukotrienes and Essential Fatty Acids*, 54; 3:183-6, 1996

Harenberg J, Giese C, Zimmermann R, Effect of dried garlic on blood coagulation, fibrinolysis, platelet aggregation and serum cholesterol levels in patients with hyperlipoproteinemia, *Atherosclerosis*, 74:247-9, 1988

Neil HAW, Silagy C, Garlic: its cardioprotective properties, *Curr Opin Lipidol*, 5:6-10, 1994

McMahon FG, Vargas R, Can garlic lower blood pressure? A pilot study. *Pharmacotherapy* 13:406-7, 1993

Santo OS, Grunwald J, Effect of garlic powder tablets on blood lipids and blood pressure. A six-month placebo-controlled double-blind study, *Brit J Clin Res* 4:37-44, 1993

Orekhov AN, Pivovarova EM, Tertov VV, Garlic powder tablets reduce atherogenicity of low density lipoprotein. A placebo-controlled double-blind study, *Nutr Metab Cardiovasc Dis*, 1996, 6:21-31

Das I, et al, Potent activation of nitric oxide synthase by garlic: a basis for its therapeutic applications, *Curr Med Res Opin*, 13: 257 63, 1995

Whelton PK, He JA, Cutler JA, et al, Effects of oral potassium on blood pressure. Meta-analysis of randomized controlled clinical trials, *J Am Med Assoc*, 227; 20:1624-32, 1997

Wester PO, Dyckner T, Magnesium and hypertension, *J Amer Coll Nutr*, 6; 4: 321-328, 1987

Classen HG, Magnesium and potassium deprivation and supplementation in animals and man: aspects in view of intestinal absorption. *Magnesium*, 3; 4-6: 257-264, 1984

Barri YM, Wingo CS, The effects of potassium depletion and supplementation on blood pressure: a clinical review, *Amer J Med Sci*, 314; 1: 37-40, 1997

Taddei S, Mattei P, Virdis A, Sudano I, Ghiadoni L, Salvetti A, Effect of potassium on vaso-dilatation to acetylcholine in essential hypertension, *Hypertension*, 223; 4: 485-490, 1994

Cappuccio FP, MacGregor GA, Does potassium supplementation lower blood pressure? A meta-analysis of published trials, *J Hypert* 9; 5: 465-473, 1991

Whelton PK, Hr J, Cutler JA, Brancati FL, Appel LJ, Follmann D, Klag MJ, Effects of oral potassium on blood pressure. Meta-analysis of randomized controlled clinical trials, *J Amer Med Assoc*, 227; 20: 1624-1632, 1997

Smith SR, Klotman PE, Svetkey LP, Potassium chloride lowers blood pressure and causes natriuresis in older patients with hypertension, *Journal American Society Nephrology*, 2; 8: 1302-1309, 1992

Fotherby MD, Potter JF, Long-term potassium supplementation lowers blood pressure in elderly hypertensive subjects, *Intern J of Clin Prac*, 621; 4: 219-222, 1997

Fotherby MD, Potter JF, Potassium supplementation reduces clinic and ambulatory blood pressure in elderly hypertensive patients, *J Hypert*, 210; 11: 1403-1408, 1992

Whelton PK, Buring J, Borhani NO, Cohen JD, Cook N, Cutler JA, et al, The effect of potassium supplementation in persons with a high-normal blood pressure. Results from phase one of the Trials of Hypertension Prevention (TOHP). Trials of Hypertension Prevention Collaborative Research Group, *Ann Epid*, 5; 2: 85-95, 1995

Khaw KT, Thom S, Randomized double-blind cross-over trial of potassium on blood pressure in normal subjects, *Lancet*, 2; 1308: 1127-1129, 1982

MacGregor GA, Smith SJ, Markandu ND, Banks RA, Sagnella GA, Moderated potassium supplementation in essential hypertension, *Lancet*, 2; *8298: 567-570, 1982*

Mountokalakis, Diuretic-induced magnesium deficiency, *Magnesium* 2:57, 1983

Altura BM, Altura BT, New perspectives on the role of magnesium in the pathophysiology of cardiovascular system, II. Experimental; aspects, *Magnesium* 4:245-71, 1985

Singh RB, Cameron EA, Relation of myocardial magnesium deficiency to sudden death in ischaemic heart disease, *Amer Heart J*, 103; 3:399-450, 1982

Parker-Pope T, Health advice that's tough to swallow: Nine helpings of fruits and veggies a day, *Wall Street Journal*, D1, April 29, 2003

Pins JJ, et al, Do whole-grain oat cereals reduce the need for antihypertensive medications and improve blood pressure control? *J Fam Pract* 51: 353-359, 2002

Suetsuna K, Maekawa K, Chen JR, Antihypertensive effects of *Undaria pinnatifida* (wakame) peptide on blood pressure in spontaneously hypertensive rats, *J Nutr Biochem*, 15:267-72, 2004

Suetsuna K, Separation and identification of angiotensin 1-converting enzyme inhibitory peptides from peptic digest of *Hizikia fusiormis* protein, *Nippon Suisan Gakkaishi*, 64:862-6, 1998

Nakano T, Hidaka H, Uchida J, et al, Hypotensive effects of wakame, *J Jpn Soc Clin Nutr* 20:92, 1998

Li GH, Le GW, Shi YH, Shrestha S, Angiotensin I-converting enzyme inhibitory peptides derived from food proteins, and their physiological and pharmacological effects, *Nutr Res* 24:469-86, 2004

Benado M, Alcantara C, Kern M, et al, Effects of various levels of dietary fructose on blood lipids of rats, *Nutr Res* 24:565-71, 2004

Merchant RE, Andre CA, Sica DA, Pilot study: Nutritional supplementation with *Chlorella pyrenoidosa* for mild to moderate hypertension, *J Am Nutraceut. Assoc*, 6; 3:33-42, 2003

Munoz SS, 'Whole grain': Food labels' new darling?, *Wall Street J*, B1, B4, Jan 12, 2005.

Skou JC, Enzymatic basis for active transport of Na+ and K+ across cell membranes, *Physiol Rev*, 45:596-617, 1965

Engler MD, et al, Flavenoid-the rich dark chocolate improves endothelial function and increases plasma epicatechin concentrations in healthy adults, *J Am Coll Nutr*, 23; 3:197-204,2004

Chiao JW, et al, Sulforaphane and its metabolite mediate growth arrest and apoptosis in human prostate cancer cells, *Int J Oncol*, 20:631-6, 2002

Maheo K, et al, Inhibition of cytochromes P-450 and induction of glutathione S-transferases by sulforaphane in primary human and rat hepatocytes, *Cancer Res*, 57; 3649-52, 1997

Kassahun K, et al, Biotransformation of the naturally occurring isothiocyanate sulforaphane in the rat: identification of phase I metabolites and glutathione conjugates, *Chem Res Toxicol*, 10; 1228-33, 1997

Ye L, Zhang Y, Total intracellular accumulation levels of dietary isothiocyantes determine their activity in elevation of cellular glutathione and induction of Phase 2 detoxification enzymes, *Carcinogenesis*, 22; 1987-92, 2000

Chen PR, Lee CC, Chang H, Tsai CE, Sesamol regulates plasminogen activator gene expression in cultured endothelial cells: a potential effect on the fibrinolytic system, *J Nutr Biochem*, 16: 59-64, 2005

Sera N, Morita K, Tokiwa H, et al, Binding effect of polychlorinated compounds and environmental carcinogens on rice bran fiber, *J Nutr Biochem*, 16: 50-58, 2005

Chapter VI

You Are Now Too Smart to Fail

Let's face it. You are a changed person now with all you have learned. You can never go back to the archaic world of drug-oriented medicine. No one can easily pull the wool over your eyes. You know more about how to heal your hypertension (and other diseases) than most doctors. But just in case you find yourself thinking none of this appeals to you, or that it's easier to do drugs, let's look at some other solutions. For you are now too smart to fail.

A Myriad of Other Solutions

Make no mistake, rare is the person who would need all the remedies in this book to heal their hypertension, and likewise rare is the person who could not heal his hypertension with any of the protocols that are contained in here. However, there are many more cures that I will continue to give you here and in the monthly inexpensive subscription *TW* newsletter, *Total Wellness*, designed to save you money while teaching you how to get progressively more independently healthy. Fortunately, rare is the person who falls outside of the range of usual causes of hypertension, yet on the flip side there are so many more ways to cure hypertension that they could not all fit in one book.

Another problem is no one knows which is the best remedy for you. However, having lived with yourself and now armed with this new knowledge, you are most likely the person best equipped to guess which remedies would be more likely to cure your hypertension. So let's be practical.

Obviously if you are a smoker, STOP. The pesticides, additives, coal tars and other chemicals in smoke damage the endothelial lining in a myriad of ways, leading to Mr. ED (*Verdecchia*). Get whatever you need in your life to make you happier or more relaxed than you are with your cigarette addiction. Do you need hypnosis? A reason to live? For every puff chews up about 100 mg of vitamin C, that you learned in Chapter II is so important to the health of the endothelial lining and for making the vasodilator, NO (nitric oxide). Check *Pain Free In 6 Weeks* for all the heart, arthritis, and other system damage that this deadly nightshade does.

Or if you have a junk food diet, getting onto a whole foods plan and doing the oil change may be all you need (Chapters V and III, respectively). If you are overweight by 20 pounds or more, a whole foods diet and oil change are the first step as well. Studies show that 80% of folks who stayed on a diet to lower their pressure were able to get off all medications (*Espeland*). But overweight also comes from cells poisoned with plasticizers that leach out of plastic food containers and wrappings, into our foods and then into our bodies. That's where your far infrared sauna comes in, for it is the only way along with weight loss that can get the plasticizers out of the body (Chapter IV). As long as the intracellular peroxisomes are poisoned with plasticizers (phthalates) some people's chemistry for weight loss (or healing anything else) is indefinitely stalled or paralyzed. They can't lose weight until the plasticizers are out (see *Detoxify or Die* for more details). And don't forget the lifesaver, Detoxamin.

Above all, never underestimate the power of getting off trans fatty acids (Chapter III). For they raise the LDL (bad) cholesterol, which raises the ADMA (Chapter II), which lowers the nitric oxide, which lets Mr. ED gallop onto the scene, ushering in among other things, hypertension (*Boger*).

Meanwhile, it has been clearly shown that vitamins, minerals, fatty acids and other nutrients are absolutely essential in staving off premature aging and degenerative diseases that you are erroneously told are "normal" consequences of aging (*Fairfield, Fletcher, Ames, Hodis, Sahyoun, Losonczy, Hu*). Don't forget that we are the generation hoodwinked by advertising that, for example, berated women for decades until they took estrogens to "prevent" heart and blood vessel diseases. Finally government-supported studies were done that duplicated what other studies had shown in the past but had been ignored. They clearly showed that women actually increase their risk of vascular disease and heart death by more than 26% by taking these estrogens derived from horse urine, and that they are actually carcinogenic, dangerously raising cancer levels for humans (*Rossouw*).

And don't fall for the ridiculous statement that you get enough nutrition from your foods and do not need nutrients. I would frankly be embarrassed for any one who would say that, as it was corrected years ago in the *Journal of the American Medical Association*. The reasons are so numerous but let's give you the highlights in a nutshell to defend yourself:
- The soils are progressively more depleted from acid rain and repeated growing of crops.
- Consequently, food measurements show that foods do not have as much nutrient value.
- The body is exposed to more pollutants than ever before in the history of the world requiring more detox nutrients.

- Plus the work of detoxifying these chemicals uses up nutrients at an unprecedented rate.
- Nutrients have been proven to change the course of chronic diseases and in fact to be the essential way to heal most diseases (*Fairfield, Fletcher, Moss, Liu, Prasad*).
- There is marked polymorphism among people, meaning that we do not all process our nutrients in our bodies the same way or at the same rate, leaving some people dependent upon nutrients for survival and health (*Rosenberg, Carson*). For example, the homocysteine that you learned about caused by the HCT blood pressure medicine, can be caused by an inborn error of metabolism in some folks. It can cause mental deficiency in children (*Carson*), or Alzheimer's, heart attack, and lots of other premature causes of death and disease if not found and corrected. It is often corrected with B vitamins, including folic acid. But some people lack the gene to properly metabolize folic acid, so they need a special form, like sublingual **Folixor** (dissolve 1 mg under your tongue) and in higher doses than normal to correct their homocysteine and thwart disease. But what a shame when it is not discovered and corrected (*Boushney*).

And worse, every drug depletes nutrients from the body, setting you up even more so for disease (*Pelton*). The sly tricks that have been pulled on the American public to convince them that drugs are the answer to every symptom and to steer them away from health-restoring nutrients have filled many books that I showed you in Chapter I. And now many people who are on a few drugs are also on a drug that is specific for the side effects caused by one of their other drugs ---- as though this new drug will somehow miraculously be devoid of any new side effects! So let's take a look at some other important nutrients plus hormones for controlling blood pressure.

Furthermore, although bear in mind I've given you lots of nutrient supplementation ideas and data here, many have also been highly successful with far less. For example, in one study they merely gave diabetics with high blood pressure the following 4 supplements:

- 200 mg magnesium oxide (cheap, only 50% absorbed)
- 30 mg zinc sulfate
- 200 mg vitamin C
- 150 mg vitamin E (looks like it probably was synthetic since they didn't designate).

They not only impressively lowered their blood pressure, but it increased their potassium (remember you can't absorb enough potassium without magnesium, which is deficient in most people). And they lowered their free radicals, so they were slowing down aging, all with only four supplements (*Farvid*). They used magnesium oxide, which means they really under-dosed them (equivalent to 100 mg/day), and the study was in diabetics, which gave them even more deficiencies to begin with than average. Yet they succeeded with an unbalanced schedule, that would inevitably create further deficiencies, plus they never measured their deficiencies of any nutrients. So don't let my enthusiastic recommendations scare you.

Coenzyme Q10

Coenzyme Q10 is likened to the spark plug in the heart muscle. It is a crucial enzyme in the mitochondria or energy factory of every endothelial (blood vessel lining) and heart muscle cell. Although the highest levels in the body are in the heart, blood vessels need it as well. In one study after just 10 weeks of 50 mg of CoQ10 twice a day, patients lowered their b.p. from an average of 165 to 145 for the top or systolic pressure. On the bottom or diastolic number they lowered it from an average of 98 to 86 (*Digiesi, Houston*). Just think what they could have accomplished with the addition of other nutrients that you have learned about here as well. For this was only one nutrient, and not necessarily the most deficient for all individuals. In other studies, after four months of CoQ10 at a daily dose of 225 mg, most patients dropped between one and three blood pressure medications. Again this was merely one nutrient, and not a package, nor was it addressing the specific deficiencies of individuals.

You learned about the potentially deadly side effects of prescription medications for hypertension in Chapter I. But as always, with natural medicine, you get good "side effects", which usually include curing or improving other seemingly (by conventional medicine standards) unrelated symptoms or diseases. CoQ10 is no exception. In one study while treating hypertension with CoQ10, there was concomitant improvement in such a serious disease as insulin resistance (*Singh*). Also called Syndrome X and metabolic syndrome (you've probably noticed multiple names emerge when medicine is really stumped with how to cure a disease), which often includes not only hypertension but diabetes that is tough to regulate, weight gain that is often tough to regulate, as well as other symptoms. Anyway, CoQ10's "coincidental" improvements don't by any means stop there, but include congestive heart failure, angina, cancer, periodontal disease, depression, chronic fatigue, and much more (*TW*).

My favorite forms are **Opti-Q-100** and **Q-Gel.** Opti-Q-100 is the liquid form that cancer studies were done on that caused regression (melting away) of breast cancers as well as metastases, at doses of less than 400 mg a day. One teaspoon provides 100 mg of coenzyme Q10. The dose, depending on your hs-CRP level (Chapter III) and other needs, would be 1/2-2 tsp. 2-3 times a day. Q-Gel is a form that has exceptionally unique water solubility, increasing absorption and giving it the highest blood levels of any form of CoQ10. In fact in some studies it tripled the doses in the blood stream compared with other types after several weeks' use, making it a superior product. The dose for the 30 mg capsule is usually in the vicinity of 1-3 capsules 2-3 times a day.

High Blood Pressure and Impotency:
The Hormone Connection

There are many reasons why it is far too common for impotency to accompany high blood pressure. (1) One nasty side effect of diuretics and other types of blood pressure medications is loss of libido or sex drive, and diminished ability to sustain or even get an erection. There are many reasons for this. First, often the very deficiencies that caused high blood pressure also overlap and cause loss of libido and *erectile dysfunction* (Oh my gosh, another Mr. ED? Actually they can both have the same causes in many cases). Magnesium deficiency that you learned about in Chapter I is a good example. It is an extremely common deficiency that is present in half of folks, or every other person. Magnesium deficiency can cause high blood pressure, fatigue, insomnia, muscle spasms, atrial fibrillation, angina, migraines, colitis, and loss of libido for starters. So it is not unusual with prescription blood pressure medications to get worsening and loss of libido and emergence of erectile dysfunction as the medicine causes further loss of magnesium and potassium.

(2) Second, as the nitric oxide synthesis gets lower that you learned about in Chapter II, it not only causes high blood pressure but loss of libido. For if you can't dilate the blood vessels, you can't get an erection. You have learned of the many things that can cause lowered NO, such as a vitamin C deficiency, especially caused by smoking. So can an undiagnosed ADMA or elevated hs-CRP, as from a tooth with smoldering infection in a root canal that has not yet given you cause for concern, but is everyday seeding dangerous bacteria into your heart and systemic blood vessels (Chapter II).

(3) A third reason why blood pressure victims also commonly have erectile dysfunction is that low testosterone or low adrenal hormone DHEA can both cause erectile dysfunction, as well as hypertension. As folks get older, and this includes women just as much as men, they tend to make less testosterone for a number of reasons (nutrient deficiencies, toxic levels of plasticizers, etc.). And **as testosterone goes down, the blood pressure tends to go up**. As well as predicting arteriosclerosis, lower testosterone predicts poor memory, prostate cancer and sexual dysfunction (impotency, poor libido), which are currently seen as mere Viagra, Cyalis or Levitra deficiencies! But you can boost testosterone in many ways, for example with your oil change that you had to do anyway for your hypertension. And you can take non-prescription **Quantum Testosterone Complex**, an extremely well tolerated combination of natural hormone precursors. This is a lot smarter approach because you'll not be taking actual testosterone to cause feedback inhibition, so

you won't turn off your natural hormone production. I have seen the laboratory results that confirm it can elevate progesterone, testosterone, DHEA and cortisol levels with its natural botanical hormone boosters.

No question, the best way to get your testosterone measured is with the **Cardiovascular Risk Panel** (MetaMetrix) which not only includes testosterone but other heart risk indicators like the most important indicator of early heart attack, the high sensitivity CRP. Also included in the **Cardiovascular Risk Panel** are insulin, fibrinogen, lipoprotein, ferritin (stored iron, a free radical initiator), vitamin E, homocysteine, lipid peroxides, RBC magnesium, sex hormone binding globulin, and coenzyme Q10, plus the standard cholesterol, HDL, LDL, and triglycerides making it unparalleled. Clearly every cardiologist in the country should be using this test, yet sadly the uninformed don't even know it exists.

Or You Can Make Your Own Testosterone

Testosterone is often thought of as just a male hormone but that's not true. We women need it as well. And when it is supplemented, there is often improvement in blood pressure, coronary risk factors, memory, decreased cancers and osteoporosis, better endurance, better mood, energy, libido, and slowed aging. A common complaint of women with low testosterone is no longer any interest in sex. But DHEA supplements have improved desire, arousal, lubrication, satisfaction and orgasm. DHEA is a major hormone of the adrenal or stress gland, and DHEA can then go on to become testosterone in the body metabolism of men and women.

DHEA is a supplement that does not require a prescription, but it requires care. Too much in a woman and she can get unwanted facial hair or acne. And anyone taking it who does not really need it can turn off their adrenal gland's normal production (by feedback inhibition as the blood stream sends the message that there is already enough DHEA present so there is no need to make any more). You really want to know your levels. A **DHEA** level, the number one hormone made by the adrenal gland, is part of the **Adrenal Stress Profile** (MetaMetrix), which also measures another adrenal hormone, cortisol, four times throughout 24-hours. It is a very easy test to do at home, because you merely collect saliva.

If the testosterone or DHEA is low, 50-100 mg of **DHEA** daily are proven to increase not only DHEA, but also the testosterone level. For DHEA (dehyroepiandrosterone), the main hormone from the adrenal or stress gland converts to testosterone in the body. The cleanest source, still containing the electrical body of light that only once living sources have, plus the most additive-free DHEA I have found is **Premier DHEA 25 mg** (Premier Research). It may improve blood pressure, depending on the individual's other deficiencies and toxicities. It may also have an extra-added benefit of improving libido. And it sure beats dying of a heart attack from Viagra® (*Shippen, Morales, Barnhart, Fogari, Kannel, Muller, Cherrier, Moffat, Hak*).

Another form of DHEA that is also from once living sources, free of toxic tag-alongs, that avoids capsules while it allows your body to take up what it needs from the skin, is **Rejuvenex Cream** (Premier Research Labs, Round Rock TX). It has absorbable DHEA 54 mg as well as pregnenolone and progesterone in merely 1/4 tsp. rubbed on the skin daily.

Would like to test your hormones without needing a prescription and have a hormone cream custom made for you? Contact **NRG Solutions** (630-853-8383) to have your salivary hormone testing kit sent and your own custom cream compounded from the results.

The Melatonin Miracle

Inside the middle of the brain is housed the pineal gland, which puts out a hormone called melatonin that is one of nature's age-reversing hormones (*Pierpaoli*). It plays not only a role in turning down aging but in reversing cancers, insomnia, jet lag, impotency and you guessed it, high blood pressure. In fact the hours between 6-9 AM are when most heart attacks occur and when the melatonin level is at its lowest. When the pineal gland grows old, it develops calcium deposits just like the heart and blood vessels do. In fact, it's considered "normal" to see a calcified pineal gland in the middle of brain x-rays. But as you learned in Chapter IV, you can even reverse this. We need the pineal gland to modulate other hormones like steroids from the adrenal and thyroid function. Yet, melatonin is also a free radical scavenger, working as well as vitamin E in protecting blood vessels. It is one of nature's most powerful antioxidants. It also can lower cholesterol, countering plaque buildup in arteries, as well as normalize blood pressure.

Melatonin is best taken at night and try not to use NSAIDs (non-steroidal anti-inflammatory drugs like Motrin, Aleve, Celebrex, Naprosyn, aspirin, etc.) because they disrupt melatonin cycling. Also beta-blockers which are commonly prescribed for high blood pressure interfere with melatonin production as well. And don't sleep with alarm clocks and other electrical apparatus within several feet of your head, nor with enough light coming into the room where you could read the headlines of a newspaper, because both of these diminish melatonin secretion which should be maximal at night when you're sleeping. The nice relaxing dose to curb insomnia that also serves as an antioxidant can be anywhere from 1-6 milligrams before bed.

Melatonin Nanoplex has 2 mg /drop, and is free of synthetic toxic tag-alongs. As well, this company specializes in keeping products solvent free, testing high-quality ingredients and then using living probiotic bacteria to nanize them to small molecular size. This serves to preserve their "body of light" which is very important in countering degeneration of our cells, so common from synthetic nutrients and hormones. Because melatonin is a strong antioxidant it has not only improved blood pressure, but reversed free radical damage in the aorta and even lowered levels of nasty amyloid deposits in the brain which lead to Alzheimer's (*Cavallo, Lahiri, Sener, Tan, Zhang*). Although rarely a complete cure for hypertension by itself, certainly a good night's sleep is a healthful start for healing any malady.

Do You Have a Hidden Thyroid Deficiency?

One of the nastiest tricks that can be played on an innocent patient is to have all the classic signs of a glandular deficiency, but the blood tests for that deficiency come out normal. Suppose you cannot lose weight, or have exhaustion, depression, constipation, or hair loss. And maybe you have high blood pressure too. You beg your doctor for a thyroid blood test, but if he is not up on the information in *Detoxify or Die*, he will trust the blood test rather than your symptoms. Well, the plasticizers that you learned about in Chapter IV can damage your thyroid function, giving you any and all these symptoms without damaging the classic blood tests used to diagnose it. "Everything looks fine, it's not your thyroid", may be your doctor's answer.

However, when folks just like this were treated with natural thyroid, 8 out of 10 normalized their blood pressure, fatigue and other symptoms. These docs called this sub-clinical hypothyroidism (*Gaby*). At least they listened to their patients and gave them the benefit of the doubt, even if they didn't know about phthalates and Iodoral. But they had a legitimate excuse, because this study was done in 1975, while a similar study was done in 1950 (*Barnes, Menof*). But you must remember that listening to the patient was much more in vogue then than it is now. Now they only treat you if your lab test is absolutely abnormal, and they don't do the correct tests to diagnose hidden causes (thyroid autoantibodies, phthalate induced-fatty acid abnormalities) to diagnose the need for a clinical trial of thyroid (*Dernellis*).

As well, a hidden thyroid deficiency can normalize elevated homocysteine in 44% of folks (*Hussein*). That shows us how inadequate the tests for thyroid is. It also points up the need for a trial of Iodoral even more (see Chapter IV) whenever there is question of adequate thyroid. Take one **Iodoral a day** for 3-6 months, while you find a doc who reads *DOD* or *TW* for the rest of your thyroid needs. And if you actually have a classic thyroid disease diagnosed, like Grave's disease, don't just rely on a prescription of synthetic thyroid.

Even just **Iodoral** and **ACES with Zinc** can potentially correct your thyroid permanently (*Vrca*). You need to correct the missing iodine/iodide as well as selenium and antioxidants so your thyroid can recover and not need to be drugged for the rest of its life. More than ever I hope you get the message that when you think something should be checked out, to always **stick to your guns**. After 35 years in medicine I've learned that most of the time a patient's suspicions are correct. So stay with your instincts.

Vitamin D for Hypertension?

I always thought that vitamin D was pretty boring. It's important for bones, the recommended daily requirement is about 400 I.U., it is added to milk, we make it from sunshine, and a deficiency causes rickets, which is rare anymore. Boy, have we been duped again!

It turns out that vitamin D receptors are in nearly every tissue of the body, especially the brain, breast, prostate and white blood cells. And recent research shows that higher vitamin D levels provide protection from diabetes, congestive heart failure, metabolic syndrome, depression, autoimmune diseases like lupus and cancers of the breast, prostate and colon, plus - - - you guessed it, high blood pressure. If that were not enough, numerous studies of all different walks of life from affluent teenagers in Boston to older hospitalized patients show that vitamin D deficiency is epidemic in anywhere from 42-93% of the population.

And if that were not bad enough, like so many other nutrients, the "normal" blood levels are much too low, while the cut-off for deficiencies is way too high. This means that blood tests either make folks look normal or like they have too much vitamin D, when in reality most are dangerously deficient. **Should the Recommended Daily Allowance or RDA really stand for Ridiculously Dangerous Advice?** For the RDA for vitamin D is 400 I.U., in spite of studies that clearly show it should be at least 10 times this or 4000 I. U. daily, which has been shown to be not only safe, but necessary.

As with other nutrients, we've been given a false sense of security in many ways such as through the "fortification" of common foods like milk via synthetic vitamins. Real vitamin D is D3 or cholecalciferol and is produced in the skin and consumed in the diet. But the one added to milk is synthetic D2, ergocalciferol, produced by irradiating fungi and is less effective and more toxic. That's why with studies that say lower levels of vitamin D are toxic or don't help, you right away want to know if they used the inferior and cheaper synthetic form, the same one food processors put in milk. For indeed there are many deleterious effects from synthetic nutrients, including hardening of arteries.

If you have resistant high blood pressure, or for that matter, depression, seizures, inflammatory conditions like arthritis, auto-immune diseases like lupus, diabetes, recurrent infections, heart failure, or even cancer, think of raising your vitamin D levels. But none of us were trained in medicine to think of vitamin D deficiency in those diseases, only for rickets. Chances are you are low, and it takes 2-6 months to correct a deficiency. In cancer, for example, vitamin D is necessary for redifferentiation (*Vieth*). Translation: making cancer cells go back to normal cell morphology (*TW*).

196

Vitamin D clearly has multiple roles in hypertension (*Hanni, Lind, Kurtz*) yet in spite of epidemic deficiencies, it is not yet routinely tested even in diseases that scream "Vitamin D deficiency", like osteoporosis. Not surprisingly, Vitamin D levels are frequently low in folks with osteoporosis, but it is rarely checked, as osteoporosis is misguidedly treated as a deficiency of Fosamax or Actonil! No wonder they fail to reach their mark of total cure. It's criminal to ignore basic body chemistry that even a high school student knows. So don't be bashful about asking for vitamin D3 levels, since the evidence for silent epidemic deficiency comes from the top journals like the *New England Journal of Medicine* and the *Journal of the American Medical Association* (*Thomas, LeBoff*).

There is no excuse for not checking your vitamin D3 level for not only hypertension, but also every disease. It's just too bad you have to be the one to think of it and ask. It should be part of your regular checkup, since vitamin D receptors are in every organ and affect far more than bone. The laboratory that in my book leads the world of medicine, Meta-Metrix, is adding a **Vitamin D** metabolite assay to their **ION Panel**. This is just one more reason why you haven't even begun to have a complete physical or blood pressure evaluation to uncover curable causes until you have had an ION Panel prescribed.

Undiagnosed Vitamin D Deficiency Masquerades as Fosamax/Actonil Deficiencies

Any woman over 45 that has been to the gynecologist or the family doc for a physical exam recently, knows how hard they're pushing Fosamax or Actonil. Aren't the claims reminiscent of the thousands of docs who for decades authoritatively told women they had to take Premarin the rest of their lives in order to stave off heart attacks and strokes? Then the news hit the fan that Premarin actually promotes both of these diseases big-time as well as lung clots, breast cancer and more. Such a deal! What selling jobs the pharmaceutical companies have done on docs who avoid learning the biochemical facts. Now the same scenario seems to be repeating itself with Fosamax/Actonil. These biphosphonates are being promoted as the only way to stop osteoporosis, when they lose their effectiveness within a couple of years, if they do work. For they are usually prescribed without the benefit of RBC minerals, fatty acids, vitamin D3 or other levels that relate directly to curing osteoporosis. And if osteoporosis has begun, then you really are coerced. Better to reverse it by reading *Pain Free In 6 Weeks*.

Since checking vitamin D in an obvious D-deficiency disease is so aptly ignored, it will be a long time before its well-proven role in hypertension is given due recognition. Nevertheless, vitamin D has many roles in hypertension because it has a direct effect on cell membranes as well as calcium transport, metabolism and excretion (*Hanni*). Also since calcium also has a direct effect on hypertension, it's difficult to separate the calcium and vitamin D effects, except that many more people are beefing up their calcium than their vitamin D. Sadly, taking extra calcium is actually hastening arteriosclerosis, especially when calcium is unbalanced. Take, for example the ridiculous recommendation by most gynecologists today for women to "prevent osteoporosis" with as much as 1500 mg of calcium a day. When the body gets this unbalanced grossly abnormal recommendation, it stuffs the excess calcium overflow into the blood vessel lining, thus actually hurrying calcification or hardening of the arteries, or arteriosclerosis as we call it.

The truth is scientists are alarmed that vitamin D deficiency in the land of plenty is grossly underestimated. Yet rarely does a physician check for it, partly because the practice guidelines do not require it. But recall, the *New England Journal of Medicine* reported that 87% of the physician "authorities" who make these rules for medicine are on the payrolls of pharmaceutical companies. Magically osteoporosis becomes a lifetime Fosamax deficiency, even though its effects dwindle after a couple of years (and is a potential carcinogen). When nutrients are recommended, it's often merely calcium. But you can take all the calcium in the world and you cannot absorb it if you don't have sufficient vitamin D. And you cannot hold calcium in the bone without correcting the other mineral deficiencies and vitamin D3.

Even scarier is that the "normal" range for vitamin D is wrong or highly aberrant. The same vitamin D levels were reported as 17% low by one lab, whereas another lab reported a low of 90% (*Binkley*). In addition, the RDA (recommended daily allowance) for all nutrients is decided upon by committees which are also manned by representatives from the pharmaceutical industries and food manufacturers as well. Many hire expensive lobbyists who work toward saving their companies money by not having to put more nutrients back into foods. How is this accomplished? By pressuring committees to accept the lowest (and usually antiquated) nutrient levels (*Chapuy, Kitch, Angell, Heaney*). Medical journals give sufficient evidence that the levels are purposely too low so food manufacturers will not look bad nor have to spend extra money fortifying foods.

So when your 25-hydroxyvitamin D3 levels do come back, insist on seeing them. If they lie within the middle of the range or higher, that may be O.K., but it won't hurt to do a 1-3 month trial of one 1000mg Vitamin D3 a day extra. If they are in the middle of the normal range or lower, take more. Most labs cite the lower end of an acceptable vitamin D level as 37.5-50 nmol/L (15-20 ng/ml). You don't want to be anywhere near this level because studies show that this **"normal vitamin D" cut-off is insufficient to allow you to absorb calcium and correct osteoporosis**. You want to be at least 86-122 nmol/L, which has been shown to provide 65% greater calcium absorption.

But unfortunately the "normal" values from labs across the country are in flux and in very little agreement as this new knowledge emerges. This brings us right back to old-fashioned clinical suspicion and a therapeutic trial. And I never feel embarrassed about a therapeutic trial that is supervised. Many important discoveries have been made this way. For example, remember Lindenbaum's classic paper in the *New England Journal of Medicine* showing that the serum B12 test is useless? He essentially gave a B12 trial (blinded so they wouldn't be branded as hypochondriacs) to older folks whose standard B12 blood tests were all in the normal range. But guess what! Many of them had significant improvement in energy, mood and brainpower. Just one more reason why the more superior B12 assessment (urinary methylmalonic acid) is used in the **ION Panel** and not the inferior serum B12.

Vitamin D cuts hip fractures by one-third. Folks over 65 years old taking 100,000 mg of vitamin D by mouth once every four months over 5 years had 33% fewer hip fractures.

This was better than Fosamax (*Trivedi*).   When Boston researchers looking at teenagers found over a third of them were deficient (*Gordon*), no wonder we have the silent epidemic of other vitamin D deficiency illnesses like fibromyalgia.   In one study of fibromyalgia victims, half of them were grossly deficient in vitamin D (*J Rheumatol*, 28: 2535-39, 2001).   In another report (*Arch Intern Med*, 160: 11 99-1203, 2000), correcting vitamin D deficiency improved fibromyalgia, chronic fatigue and depression.   But who knows this?

Did you ever wonder why you have more colds in the winter?   One reason is because when there's not as much sunlight, vitamin D metabolism dwindles, but is needed by the white blood cells to fight off infection.   That's another reason there's more congestive heart failure, multiple sclerosis, rheumatoid arthritis, and heart attacks, during this season.   In the winter with less sunlight available and more indoor activity, vitamin D levels reach their lowest, accentuating the silent epidemic of undiscovered vitamin D deficiency.

In addition, we need vitamin D for all sorts of other important things like differentiation of breast cancers and other cancers.   Differentiation can make cancer cells revert back to normal cells, and is the process that keeps them from becoming cancerous to begin with.   And even if you do get breast cancer, for example, vitamin D makes the chemotherapy work better against the cancer cell, while at the same time protecting the normal cells from dying from chemotherapy.   If you have any cancer or bone problems such as arthritis, fractures, osteoporosis, osteopenia, or fibromyalgia, insist on a vitamin D assay.

Think Vitamin D for Disease:
Diabetes, Hypertension, Cancer, MS, and More

Vitamin D has many roles in the regulation of not only blood pressure, but insulin metabolism, triglycerides and much more, which can indirectly effect **hypertension** *(Hanni, Lind, Kurtz, Trived, Ravid, Holick)*. You know that there is a current epidemic of diabetes in not only adults but also children. And diabetes is closely tied to developing hypertension as well accelerated aging and death. But how many physicians know that our hidden epidemic of vitamin D deficiency is partly the cause? One of the most commonly prescribed medications for diabetes, generic metformin (brand names include Glucovance, Metaglip, and Glucophage), only improves insulin sensitivity by 13%. Compare this with folks who were given vitamin D and improved their insulin sensitivity 21%. **In other words natural vitamin D helps diabetics better than the expensive prescription medications loaded with side effects.** And for folks that already have higher levels of vitamin D on board, their insulin sensitivity was boosted to 60% better. Once more it would appear that synthetic drugs from the laboratory couldn't improve upon God's chemistry.

No wonder the pharmaceutical, insurance, and medical communities do not want you measuring vitamin levels and curing diseases. No wonder they shun covering nutrient levels as well as taking nutrients, even if recommended by a physician, since then they would not sell a lifetime of drugs, yielding outrageous profits. No wonder medicine has taken a quantum leap, from drug-driven medicine to genetic engineering and counseling. Conveniently, they totally bypassed the molecular biochemistry of how diseases are caused and cured. This is why the current system, aside from emergency treatments, is essentially chronic, non-curative, ineffective, and the most costly medical care in the world, without a commensurate improvement in health.

Of course diabetics have more infections than most people do partly because the white blood cell has receptors for vitamin D that must be filled in order to fight off bacteria, viruses and protozoa. If these vitamin D receptors on the surface of the white blood cells don't carry enough vitamin D, they don't work to fight infection. And diabetics have a notoriously higher level of infections. Likewise most diabetics are more prone than the average person to high blood pressure and heart disease and you need sufficient vitamin D for the endothelial and heart receptors to control these diabetic side effects (*Vasquez , Zittermann*).

Vitamin D sufficiency can be assessed via the **ION Panel** (MetaMetrix). My preferred supplement source to correct your deficiency while you get on a healthier whole foods diet would be 1-3 Carlson's **Vitamin D3 1000** I. U. daily with your other nutrients. Remember to reduce it when you take Cod Liver Oil and multiples that also contain vitamin D. It's best to have your doctor measure it. And recall that vitamin D works better in association with multiple minerals that include calcium. Carlsons' **Cod Liver Oil** contains 500 mg of vitamin D per teaspoon and 1250 mg of vitamin A. Their natural **1000 mg Vitamin D3** also has 1600 mg of vitamin A. So when tallying up your total daily levels of nutrients you can aim anywhere from 2000-8000 I. U. of vitamin D daily and easily 10,000 mg or more of vitamin A, remembering to always keep the levels in the range recommended by your gynecologist if you are pregnant.

And having a low vitamin D level in muscles most likely contributes to the painful and deadly muscle disease, rhabdomyolysis, a lethal side effect caused by the statin cholesterol-lowering drugs. As well, multiple studies show higher vitamin D levels lower your risk for prostate, breast and colon cancers. Calcitriol, the most potent metabolite of vitamin D, suppresses the major trigger for inflammation TNFa (tumor necrosis factor, for which the dangerous new drugs like Enbrel® and Remicade® are prescribed). But inflammation isn't limited to arthritis, for it is the basic underlying mechanism for developing arteriosclerosis with coronary and carotid artery diseases as well as peripheral vasculitis. Clearly vitamin D has a role to play in many of the mechanisms whereby diabetes gets worse, ushering in tragic blindness, debilitating heart disease, cancers, nerve damage, cataracts, hypertension, and early death (*Vasquez, Zittermann*).

The good news is that improving your vitamin D levels can dramatically slow all this down. And don't forget that vitamin D works in multiple ways not only in diabetes, but all other diseases and is one of the hidden stumbling blocks where folks will never get well until someone thinks of it and raises the dose. It is foolish to fail to check and correct vitamin D levels in anyone before sentencing them to a lifetime of osteoporosis drugs like Fosamax or Actonil. Currently the evidence really indicates that vitamin D levels should be checked in every disease and well people are no exception. Even researchers at the Massachusetts General Hospital in Boston found that correcting unsuspected vitamin D deficiencies in folks with multiple sclerosis vastly reduced the worsening of multiple sclerosis to the wheelchair stage. I wonder what a 3-6 month trial of vitamin D will do for your blood pressure?

Vitamin K Rips Calcium from Arteries

Now that we have had over a decade of the insane recommendation of huge amounts of calcium to prevent osteoporosis, plus fortification of junk "fruit" drinks with calcium, how do we get this age-accelerating, hypertension-producing calcium out of arteries? In addition, as more and more folks are getting ultrafast heartscans and finding calcifications in their coronary arteries, heart valves, the aorta or the carotids (neck vessels leading to the brain), the question comes up about what you're going to do about them. How do we remove these calcifications from the arteries?

For starters, would you believe that **vitamin K is one of the tools for pulling calcifications out of arteries?** If you think like I used to, vitamin K just conjures up images of making blood clot. But in reality, it also is responsible for keeping blood from abnormally clotting (*Ronden*), yet it does a ton more like inhibiting cancer and metastases (*Jancin*). Vitamin K transforms blood proteins (through carboxylation) into **proteins with claws that can hang onto calcium** so that it can be moved around in the body to the proper places. Proteins that don't have enough vitamin K "claws" can't "get a grip" (pardon the pun, I couldn't control myself) on minerals to control where they go. So without properly carboxylated or "gripping" proteins, calcium trickles out of bones and into places where it doesn't belong, like arteries and other soft tissues such as tendons, ligaments and bones.

Wow, how interrelated vitamins D and K are! Osteocalcin is one of the proteins that requires vitamin K to work and to enable vitamin K to regulate calcium. When there is not enough vitamin K, no matter how much calcium is given to build bones, calcium still leaches out of bones and teeth. It then ends up calcifying or hardening our arteries in the heart (coronaries), in neck vessels that lead to the brain (carotids), and even in the main artery that leads from the heart to the rest of the body, the aorta. This is similar to what happens when there is not enough vitamin D. Now you can begin to understand why studies show that **folks who have osteoporosis** (which is definitely not limited to women) don't die from broken bones; they **die from increased numbers of heart attacks**. And a stroke (the 3rd most common cause of death) is merely the brain's version of a heart attack. Reminiscent of the vitamin D debacle again, isn't it?

Also when calcium is not properly regulated, hypertension is a common result as well as Alzheimer's and inflammatory arthritis. For you see, vitamin K does even more than regulate calcium. It inhibits cytokines like IL-6 that create inflammation and trigger the E4 proteins that are a diagnostic tip-off that someone is going to have Alzheimer's. As well, vitamin K has dramatically cut cancer metastases and more than doubled survival. Once again, you can appreciate how interlocked many of the body mechanisms are. When we fail to find and fix the underlying causes of even one symptom, like high blood pressure, we set ourselves up for getting cancer, osteoporosis, and other diseases.

Now back to the calcified arteries and heart valves; calcification is just as dangerous as fatty buildup in arteries. Knowing the role of vitamin K, some researchers created animals with hardening of the arteries with a special heart attack diet. Some of the animals were given vitamin K and others were given vitamin E. After just a few weeks, **vitamin K reduced the level of unwanted calcium in the aorta** from 17.5

mcg/mg to 1 mcg/mg, while adding vitamin E reduced it even more (*Seyama*). Furthermore, **vitamins K and E drastically reversed heart valve damage from the heart attack diet**. What would adding Detoxamin have done?

Obviously you need a lot more than just vitamin K and you know how to get the **Cardio/ ION Panel** in order to identify your remaining deficiencies. As well, it's important to reduce your levels of stockpiled heart-damaging chemicals with the **Far Infrared sauna** and the accelerated heavy-metal detox protocol (Chapter IV), preferably with Detoxamin. You also learned about using vasodilating and plaque reducing **L-Arginine Powder** (Chapter II). Now would be a good time for you and your physician to consider adding vitamin K to your regimen, and he is especially needed if you are on any blood thinners like heparin or Coumadin (generic warfarin, originally and still is a rat poison), which cause osteoporosis among other symptoms. An excellent source of vitamin K is Thorne's **Vitamin K2** 1 mg, which does require a prescription. **Super K with K2** (Life Extension Foundation, lef.com) has 9 mg K1 in addition to the 1 mg K2 and does not require a prescription. A very promising non-prescription source is 15 mg K2 in capsules (from a Canadian company, AOR) called **Peak K2** at 1-877-402-5450 or y2khealthanddetox.com .

If you were to use high doses of K2 as with 15 mg of Peak K2, you should do so with strict guidance by your physician, measuring fibrinogen, CRP, and more via the Cardio/ION Panel. The RDA (recommended daily allowance) for vitamin K is 400 mcg (0.4mg). So a dose of 15 mg is enormously higher. However, before your physician panics, I would remind him that many studies have been safely done with 45-

90 mg of vitamin K for prevention or treatment of osteoporosis as well as liver cancer prevention in folks with viral hepatitis (*Habu, Asakura, Orimo*). During those studies they looked at the standard blood clotting tests in order to guard against any hypercoagulability and found none.

Because vitamin K is not stored in the body, and because healthy intestinal bacteria (which are often killed by antibiotics and junk food diets) normally form it, most people are low. I'll cover lots more about K2 and other ways of reversing arterial calcifications in upcoming *TW* issues for you, and eventually map out a whole program for reversing arteriosclerosis, which is beyond the focus of this book. For now make sure you have a healthy gut that can make vitamin K. If you have any symptoms of gas, bloating, pain, indigestion, diarrhea, constipation, blood or mucus, have your doctor include in your work-up a **Comprehensive Stool** test (Doctor's Data). This is in my estimation after 35 years in active medical practice the best assay available for finding unwanted bugs in the gut that are stalling healing. And it can indicate whether you have enough pancreatic enzymes in order to absorb your fat-soluble vitamins, D, K, E, A, B-carotene and CoQ10. This stool test by Doctor's Data is far superior to any hospital assay that I have seen. To learn more about naturally healing the gut, read *No More Heartburn*. By all means, steer clear of heartburn medications, as by turning off acid and other functions they are another fast ticket to accelerated aging.

Dissolve the Cholesterol Right Off the Vessel

Wouldn't it be great if we could reverse some of the changes in our aging blood vessels? How about something that would dissolve the old cholesterol off the blood vessel wall? Well, remember **PhosChol** that you learned was so important in the membrane sandwich in Chapter III? Phosphatidylcholine has the unique ability to also pull cholesterol off artery walls (*Samochowiec, Howard, Stafford, Yechiel, Bar*). That's right, it also reverses the arteriosclerotic changes of aging. One particular body enzyme, LCAT (Lecithin: cholesterol acyltransferase), accomplishes just that. It exchanges lecithin (which is partly phosphatidylcholine) for cholesterol and transports cholesterol from its storage site on vessel walls to the bile where it is excreted and serves a different function to emulsify or digest fats for proper body chemistry (*Gunderman*).

Now we are starting to really accumulate a number of items that will strengthen vessel walls and make them more cholesterol-proof. As well, we have amassed a number of things that will actually dissolve the plaque off from vessel walls like vitamin K2, arginine, phosphatidylcholine, EDTA in the form of a rectal suppository, Detoxamin, and oral EDTA complexed with specially well-absorbed phosphatidyl choline in the form of DetoxMax Plus, and the macrobiotic diet (Chapters II, II, III, IV, V). As well glucosamine sulfate, silicon, boron, MSM and other things are crucial in strengthening the matrix of the blood vessel wall and its electrical activity. Restoration of other nutrients and continuation of your daily Detox Enema and Detox Cocktail round out the program (Chapter II). Addition of a Nanobac program may be necessary for some (*TW*). You are beginning to appreciate that there is a nearly endless array of possibilities, and future *TW* and books will provide much more details. For now let's see how we could incorporate some of the more likely and easier cures into a manageable program for you.

Unknown Disease, DVT, Kills Over 200,000 Each Year

Would you believe there is a condition that is totally preventable that kills more people a year than the combination
of breast cancer deaths (41,000), AIDS deaths (15,000), and
fatal auto accidents (43,000)? In fact, you can even add the
epidemic deaths from prostate cancer and still this condition
kills more people than all of these together. The sad fact is it
is rarely diagnosed and usually is missed, even after folks
are dead. There is very little education instructing folks how
to avoid it, even though there was a leadership conference
devoted to it over two years ago sponsored by the American
Public Health Association and in which Harvard Medical
School professors participated (*Goldhaber*).

Over 600,000 Americans suffer from this condition every
year and if they don't die from it, they can have serious
complications that can eventually cause death. In a national
survey, 74% of adults had never heard of it and over 57%
were unable to name any risk factors. Furthermore over 95%
surveyed reported their physician had never discussed this
medical condition with them. Other studies showed that
this silent epidemic is practically ignored by the medical
profession. Part of the reason is that 50% of the people don't
even have any early symptoms before they get the serious or
fatal event. One study showed 71% of patients with it did
not receive any prophylactic medication within 30 days of
diagnosis.

The condition? DVT, deep vein thrombosis. Clots that form
in blood vessels, usually in the deep vessels of the legs, and
either go to the lungs (pulmonary embolism), brain (stroke),
or heart (heart attack). They can also go to the eye resulting

in sudden blindness. The risk factors include increasing age, and prolonged immobility like sitting on a plane or in a car or at a computer for hours without getting up. The heavier you are the more you compress the vessels in the legs, which in turn slows down blood circulation making you more likely to clot. Having any form of cancer (past or present) or any of its treatments, recent or former major surgery, and accidents, especially with fractures of the pelvis, hips or legs, make someone even more vulnerable. Likewise, many medications, fast food diets, artificial joints, hidden teeth root infections and much more increase vulnerability. The chances of these sudden fatal clots forming are increased by being overweight, having varicose veins, congestive heart failure, anything artificial inside blood vessels like catheters and stents, new heart valves and any vascular surgery, as well as inflammatory bowel disease, kidney disease called nephrotic syndrome, plus drugs like birth control pills, hormone replacement pills for menopause, wearing tight clothes, and more.

But hold on. One more agent is very potent in inducing clots, but is rarely mentioned in medicine. In fact this whole symposium devoted to DVT missed it as well: environmental chemicals. As I showed in *Detoxify or Die* and *Total Wellness*, common everyday chemicals, from diesel exhaust to cleansers are often used to induce hypercoagulability in laboratory animals. Luckily special non-prescription enzymes can inhibit this dangerous clot formation.

The symptoms of DVT (deep vein thrombosis) can range from nothing to mild or severe tenderness in a leg or arm. Or there may just be a mysterious pain, or mere swelling, or a sudden discoloration or redness or any of the above in any combination. If the clot goes to the lungs it produces unexplained shortness of breath, chest pain or sudden palpitations or arrhythmia, sudden anxiety and/or sweating and often coughing up blood. Blood thinners are the treatments in a medical facility. But you can do much more in preventing this with many agents. I especially advise these if you know you're trying to go on a long trip where prolonged sitting is necessary.

NSC-24™ Beta Glucan Circulatory Formula is one excellent prophylaxis. It contains beta-1,3/1,6-glucan, an extract from the yeast, Saccharomyces, cell wall which boosts the immune system in multiple ways and is so potent that it has been able to decrease plaque accumulation in arterial walls. As well, it contains another plaque and unwanted clots discourager, ascorbic acid (vitamin C) and the clot-dissolving enzyme bromelain, plus coenzyme Q10, chelates of magnesium and potassium as well as the vessel wall strengthening amino acids, lysine and proline. Use 2-3, three or four times a day depending on how severe you suspect that your total risk factors are.

It does more. It is also useful for preventing infections after surgery or multiple traumas, lowering the risk from 30% down to less than 5%. Since clots and infections are common side effects of surgery, this does double duty. This sure beats all of the nasty side effects of taking antibiotics, especially since many of the new hospital bugs are already resistant to them. And when combined with antibiotics, it improves their effectiveness. As well, it has anti-viral and anti-fungal properties and speeds wound healing. In *TW*, I told you about the strong anti-cancer effects of beta glucan as well its boosting of cytokines like natural killer cells, and it has even caused tumor regression (melting away of cancers). The pineapple-derived enzyme bromelain has anti-cancer properties as well as clot-busting (*Batkin*).

If you consider yourself at higher risk or want to protect yourself with increased clot-preventing power, you need to add additional clot-busting enzymes (*Braga, Carratu, Mazzonie, Fujita, Okamoto, Sumi, Ohkura, Wang, Rogers*). My favorite four are Nattokinase, Boluoke, Wobenzyme and Serrapeptase. Chose either one, take it as 2-4 capsules three times a day, between meals. An added bonus is that enzymes can improve hypertension as well as lessen the chances of deep vein thrombosis (*Fujita*).

Potent enzymes can do more than dissolve early clots and prevent them from forming further. They are so potent that they fight their way into slimy proteins called biofilms that bacteria secrete around themselves like a suit of armor, making them invisible to the immune system. Once potent enzymes have dissolved off this suit of armor, the immune system and antibiotics are enormously empowered to now kill the bugs much more easily. This is especially important in areas where there is already too much congestion and poor blood supply or too much circulation-inhibiting inflammation. Areas like the prostate gland, urinary bladder, ovaries, sinuses, or teeth roots as well as any infectious conditions like pneumonia or bronchitis are much more effectively treated when enzymes dissolve their way through inflammation and clear the path for antibiotics (*Braga, Carratu, Mazzonie*). So use enzymes to increase the potency of antibiotics and chemotherapy, since they dissolve not only clots but the protective suit of armor that bugs and cancer cells secrete around themselves (see *Wellness Against All Odds* and

TWs for cancer directions which are beyond the scope of this book).

Although the subject of this book is not cancer, I'd like to make sure that you understand how paramount the health of your blood vessels is to healing everything, including cancer. As I have shown (and referenced) in past *TW* issues, insulin given along with chemotherapy fools cancer cells into becoming gluttons for chemotherapy drugs. Sometimes cancer cells take in as much as 16 times the amount of chemo that the normal healthy cells do. This is wonderful because it concentrates the nasty chemo on killing the cancer cells and minimizes the dose of chemotherapy to normal healthy cells. This is extremely important because all chemotherapy eventually causes cancer, so you really want to concentrate it in the cancer cells and not in the rest of the body. As well, using insulin along with chemotherapy to concentrate it in the cancer cells means that you need less chemotherapy, so it's less dangerous to the body as well as cheaper. Likewise this insulin potentiated therapy also improves the sensitivity of tumors to irradiation. They die more easily and at lower, safer doses, with less side effects to the victim. But, if there is not enough nitric oxide in the blood vessels (and you are now an expert in that from earlier chapters), the insulin-potentiated killing of cancer cells is negated (*Jordan*). It doesn't work. The bottom line is, you need very healthy blood vessels and a good supply of arginine if you are fighting off cancers, or any disease. The basics that you learned here apply to every disease you ever had and will ever get. So never hesitate to refer back here and refresh your memory if you get stuck with some disease in the future. If you need more information on the huge variety of

214

treatments available for cancers, check *TW* 1999-present, and I have personalized scheduled phone consultations.

Meanwhile, deep vein thrombosis is much more prevalent, underdiagnosed, and immediately dangerous than hypertension, but equally preventable. In fact, you have total control. I hope you will reread this short section so that it becomes indelibly imprinted in your mind that silent blood clots are major killers when we do not adequately protect and fortify our blood vessels.

Wouldn't It Be Powerful
If We Could Combine a Few of These?

Now we are getting into some exciting power for reversal of the number one cause of death. You know that the **Far Infrared Sauna** is indispensable for getting rid of plasticizers, pesticides, and the myriad of other nasty chemicals that damage blood vessels and have no other way out of the body. Then we have the inexpensive indispensable detoxifier of heavy metals and unwanted calcifications, **Detoxamin.** This nightly rectal suppository version of the IV EDTA chelation drug can in many cases reverse high blood pressure, arteriosclerosis, angina, coronary calcifications, claudication, and a host of other symptoms. The other product that you may be interested in, **DetoxMax Plus,** although it is non-prescription, to assure your safety, manufacturers insist you get it by prescription or from your doctor. It is an interesting combination of oral phosphatidylcholine connected to EDTA in a lyophilized form that penetrates cells, is incredibly easy to take, and has given additional improvement in recalcitrant conditions (Chapter IV).

For speedier relief from serious hypertension, for example, there is nothing wrong with using your nutrients, far infrared sauna, **Detoxamin** and **DetoxMax Plus**. But only if you have excellent medical supervision and keep a tight eye on mineral losses via **RBC Minerals** (from MetaMetrix), which is also part of the ION Panel, and also part of the Cardio/ION. But you needn't have ordered the whole enchilada, but merely the minerals for monitoring mineral loss every 3-6 months. And remember to take trace minerals, via **IntraMin**, which includes obscure minerals for which we have no measurement yet.

I cannot stress enough however, how important it is to have your doctor read this book and to be a part of your decision-making team. For any chelation, IV, oral, or rectal, is going to also deplete good minerals. You must have someone periodically monitoring your loss of minerals so that you can keep up with their restoration. No matter how diligent you think you are, usually there are serious deficiencies that have developed after a while. For example, manganese (not to be confused with magnesium) can become very depleted, but if you are not measuring the RBC minerals, you'll never know. What happens when it is low? A myriad of things. Manganese is crucial in the mitochondrial SOD (superoxide dismutase). What does this mean? It means that without enough manganese, when the plasticizers or phthalates elevate peroxides inside the energy factory, there's nothing there to sop them up. The result is destruction of your mitochondria that translates into baffling chronic fatigue, leaving your doc convinced you are a hypochondriac.

More importantly, if you are chelating to bring your blood pressure down, but are not correcting your manganese, a deficiency of manganese leads to high blood pressure (*Kalea*), so it becomes the vicious cycle. You learned in Chapter II how important magnesium is for curing hypertension in some people. But magnesium cannot adequately work without enough manganese. So the bottom line is keep a regular check on your minerals, especially during chelation.

Putting It All Together

You have an incredible array of possible cures for your hypertension. Where do you begin? How many do you use? If the pressure is up, start with 4 stalks of organic celery a day and a whole foods diet (Chapter V) and the oil change (in Chapter III and even more detail in *Detoxify or Die*). Get an **ION Panel**, (or the best bargain and most complete test, the **Cardio/ION**) to assess the nutrient deficiencies that are contributing to your hypertension. In the meantime start 600 mg of magnesium (not oxide, for it is the least well absorbed form), using any sources in Chapter I. Also include one scoop of **L-Arginine Powder** (Chapter II). The majority of uncomplicated hypertensives will normalize within this large range of potential therapies.

Diet changes, and in fact just the word "diet" itself, can be pretty scary. But bear in mind that since most diseases take years of indiscretion before they finally manifest themselves, it makes sense for us to moderate. You can eat a healthful whole foods plan 95% of the week, and go out and have a great time with your friends when you celebrate once a week or so. It's what you eat 95% of the time that counts, not the occasional splurge. So just because you "got away" with the splurge a few times should not be a signal to let down your guard permanently. In this way you can avoid backsliding and suffering needless symptoms. For scientific evidence clearly confirms that food choices have a major bearing on health, causing well over a third of all disease.

If your pressure is not normal within a month, begin your Far Infrared Sauna and reread the Accelerated Heavy Metal Detox protocol (Chapter IV). For elevated mercury (and other toxins) is one of many risk factors for fatal heart attack, doubling the risk for having an attack and tripling the risk for death by a heart attack (*Salonen*). Mercury also increases the levels of antibodies against oxidized LDL and increases blood pressure by other mechanisms (*Sorensen*). In fact it looks like onboard mercury is a more potent risk factor for heart attacks than is smoking. And I say onboard as opposed to merely elevated mercury, because these high risk folks were often only in the highest part of the "normal" range for mercury in order to have twice the risk of heart attack (*Circulation* 102; 22: 2677-79, Nov. 28, 2000).

Getting Started

Some handy nutrients to get you started, in order of need for many, with their common daily dose ranges follow. The total daily doses shown should be spread over 2-3 two doses, which makes them more useful and manageable. On the flip side, you could spread one day's worth of nutrients over 2-3 days if you are super sensitive. The nutrients can be obtained from most of the individual companies or collectively from **NEEDS** (1-800-634-1380), which keeps most of the companies' products on hand and has been supplying our patients and readers for over a quarter of a century.

Magnesium source (choose one for 400-600 mg/day):

- Natural Calm 200 mg powder, Peter Gillham's, 1-888-800-1180, 2-3 tsp/d
- Magnesium Citrate 166 mg caps (Metabolic Maintenance), NEEDS, 1-800-634-1380
- Magnesium Chloride 85 mg/cc, Pain & Stress Center, 1-800-669-CALM
- Magnesium Chloride Solution 200 mg/cc (Rx required), Windham Pharmacy, 1-518-734-3033

Detox Cocktail (once or twice a day):

- R-Lipoic, intensivenutrition.com, 1-800-333-7414, 1-2 per DC
- Ultrafine Ascorbic Acid Powder, Klaire Labs, 1-800-533-7255, ½-2 tsp
- Recancostat (Integrative Therapeutics), NEEDS, 1-800-634-1380, 400-800 mg per DC

Necessary nutrients:

- Cod Liver Oil, carlsonlabs.com, 1-800-323-4141, 1 tsp daily
- Liquid Multiple Minerals, Carlson, 1-800-323-4141, 1-2 twice a day
- PhosChol 900, nutrasal.com 1-800-364-4416, 1 tsp or 3 caps daily
- Heartbeat Elite, carlson.com, 1-800-323-4141, 1-4 a day _or_
- Super 2 Daily, carlsonlabs.com, 1-800-323-4141, 1-2 a day
- Q-Gel CoQ10 w/carnitine, NEEDS 1-800-634-1380, 2 twice a day
- L-Arginine Powder, Carlson, 1-800-323-4141, ½-1 tsp twice a day

Other important nutrients:

- ACES with Zinc, carlsonlabs.com, 1-800-323-4141, 1 a day
- Vitamin D3 1000 I. U., carlsonlabs.com, 1-888-234-5656, 1-2 a day
- Acetyl L-Carnitine, jarrow.com, 1-800-726-0886, 1-2 twice a day
- E-Gems Elite, carlsonlabs.com, 1-800-323-4141, 1-2 a day
- IntraMin, druckerlabs.com, 1-972-881-2344, 1-2 tbs./d
- Nutra Support Joint, carlsonlabs.com, 1-888-234-5656, 1-2 twice a day

Extra minerals (one a day, especially after chelating):

- Chelated Manganese 20 mg, carlsonlabs.com, 1-800-323-4141
- Chelated Chromium 200 mcg, carlsonlabs.com, 1-800-323-4141
- Moly B, carlsonlabs.com, 1-800-323-4141
- Chelated Zinc 30 mg, carlsonlabs.com, 1-800-323-4141 _or_
- Zinc Balance (if need to correct copper, too), jarrow.com, 1-800-726-0886
- Vanadyl Factors, jarrow.com, 1-800-726-0886
- Selenium 200mcg, carlsonlabs.com, 1-800-323-4141
- Iodoral (Optimox), Belmar Pharmacy, 1-303-763-5533
- Cogimax, Optimox, 1-800-223-1601
- Boron 3mg, pureencapsulations.com, 1-800-753-2277

Detox:

- Far Infrared Sauna, hightechhealth.com, 1-800-794-5355
- Alkaline Water Machine, hightechhealth.com, 1-800-794-5355
- Detoxamin, microzyme@mindpring.com, 1-877 656-4553
- DetoxMax Plus, bioimmune.com, 1-888-663-8844
- Medicardium, Bio Botanical, 1-800-775-4140
- Captomer, (Thorne), NEEDS, 1-800-634-1380
- Chemet, Rx any pharmacy (but over-priced)

Labs:

- RBC Mineral Panel, MetaMetrix, 1-800-221-4640
- Fatty Acids blood test, metametrix.com, 1-800-221-4640
- ION Panel (contains all above), MetaMetrix, 1-800-221-4640
- Cardiovascular Risk Panel, MetaMetrix, 1-800-221-4640
- Cardio/ION Panel (contains all above and more), metametrix.com, 1-800-221-4640
- ADMA test, metametrix.com, 1-800-221-4640
- 8-OHdG (part of ION Panel), MetaMetrix, 1-800-221-4640
- Nutrient & Toxic Elements 24-hr urine, MetaMetrix, 1-800-221-4640
- Adrenal Stress Profile, metametrix.com, 1-800-221-4640
- Comprehensive Stool, Doctor's Data, 1-800-323-2784

So go over these with your doctor and decide how much of the program for starters you might need. You have many options from 4 stalks of celery a day to the most life-saving detoxification protocols.

Rationing of Health Care is Here

With all these great cures that you are learning about, I bet you were as naïve as I was in thinking that medicine would also enthusiastically embrace them. *Au contraire*, in fact they are moving in the exact opposite direction and rationing what little non-drug care they give. As I showed you in Chapter I from top medical journals, medical care is dominated by the pharmaceutical industry. There is little interest in curing folks and getting them off the very drugs that fuel the economy.

Move Over Dr. Kevorkian,
The AMA Recommends Euthanasia for the Faithful

More medical articles are showing that medicine is increasingly approaching euthanasia. This year a medical journal stated "Not infrequently, Christian patients and families provide religious justification for an insistence on aggressive medical care near the end of life." This article in an AMA (American Medical Association) journal ended with instructions for physicians to help patients reach "appropriate limits to life-sustaining treatment" (*Brett*). **Translation: Doctors, don't let Christian patients' religious beliefs keep you from playing God and telling them how long they can live.** This is part of the planned rationing of health care, because frankly we cannot afford it the way it is going now.

Can you believe an AMA journal is directing physicians to ignore Christians' wanting to do everything possible to live? Especially when you have learned that 99% of medicine is drug-driven and fills the coffers of the pharmaceutical industry at your risk. Meanwhile, the majority of physicians never do the most rudimentary biochemical analyses that you've learned about here to find the actual causes and cures of your symptoms, so you won't need death-promoting drugs.

I think I speak for you, too, when I say I don't want any group of physicians unknowledgeable in the molecular biochemistry of how to healthfully reverse disease telling me how long I can live. They want to tell you and I when it's time to stop treatments and pull the plug, when they have not a clue of what is necessary to "heal the impossible"!

I suspect you want the best form of life-saving medicine for yourself and your loved ones that I do. The new gatekeepers over your longevity (who are assuming the role of God) are the very guys who don't come to courses on nutritional, environmental and toxicologic medicine nor molecular biochemistry. They do not read books like this one. They never ever think of ordering bare minimum your red blood cell minerals and fatty acids much less anything else that could save your life. Remember the *Journal of the American Medical Association* papers that showed that in the medical mecca of Boston, 95% of doctors failed to even order the most rudimentary and grossly inferior serum magnesium test, and this is in patients many of whom died for lack of it.

Most physicians do not even know what is in an ION Panel (ask them). They for the most part rely on (1) standard blood tests (commonly called a chemical profile which looks at your liver, kidney enzymes, a few electrolytes, a blood count and indicators that are rarely abnormal until you have something serious like metastatic cancer), and (2) the latest pharmaceutical drugs, none of which heal, but merely mask symptoms while you continue to worsen and develop new diseases.

These Are Definitely Not the Guys Who Should Tell Us When to "Pull the Plug"

Even more frightening is the front page *Wall Street Journal* article showing **that non-physician hospital and insurance employees are now playing the most important role in the rationing of health-care by deciding who gets what treatments paid for** (*Anand*). This is downright scary. You now have low wage, non-medical, poorly trained folks who do not know you who are hired by the hospital or insurance company to make the decision of how much life-sustaining therapy you can have. The turnover in this type of job dealing with unhappy customers assures even poorer training of new recruits. This is scary rationing of healthcare. And even through they can practice medicine without a license, you cannot sue them (*TW* 2005).

You had better keep getting yourself progressively smarter and healthier, for your sake and those you love. That is what we designed the monthly *TW* newsletter, *Total Wellness*, for 16 years ago. And for Pete's sake never give up or assume something is incurable if you haven't at least had an **ION Panel** complete with expert interpretation and then gone on to have the provocation heavy-metal test! (see Sources for interpretations if needed). For these two are guaranteed to give more helpful information on how to heal the impossible than the standard tests which leave your doc saying, "Everything looks fine" and then sentencing you to a lifetime of symptoms-suppressing, side effect-laden drugs.

Fortunately another article in the same journal showed that folks, who request clinical services like laboratory tests, usually get them (*Kravitz*). They did state also that folks who ask for tests, specialist referrals, or particular prescriptions, but especially specialty tests, make doctors very uncomfortable. Isn't that just too bad? The moral of the story is thousands of years old: **ask and you shall receive** (*Matt 7:7*).

If you would like some places where your doctor (and you) could learn more about this type of medicine, have him contact:

- The Institute for Functional Medicine
  for excellent physician symposia, courses, books, tapes
  functionalmedicine.org, 1-800-228-0622 or fax 1-253-853-6766
- The American Environmental Health Foundation
  for physician symposia, books, less toxic products, medical care
  Aehf.com or 1-800-428-2343
- *Total Wellness* monthly subscription newsletter by this author,
  public lectures, books, radio, TV, physician lectures, personal phone
  consultations and/or laboratory interpretations
  prestigepublishing.com or 1-800-846-6687

Product Sources (also see "Putting It All Together"):

- Opti-Q-100, Phillips Nutritionals, 1-800-514-5115
- Q-Gel, NEEDS, 1-800-634-1380
- Testosterone Complex, prlabs.com, 1-800-370-3447
- DHEA, prlabs.com, 1-800-370-3447
- Rejuvenex Cream, prlabs.com, 1-800-370-3447
- Custom compounded hormones, NRG Solutions, 1-630-853-8383

- Melatonin Nanoplex, prlabs.com, 1-800-370-3447
- Comprehensive Stool, Doctor's Data, 1-800-323-2784
- Far Infrared Sauna, hightechhealth.com, 1-800-794-5355
- ION Panel, metametrix.com, 1-800-221-4640
- Adrenal Stress Profile, metametrix.com, 1-800-221-4640
- Cardio/ ION Panel, metametrix.com, 1-800-221-4640
- Vitamin D3 1000 I. U., carlsonlabs.com, 1-888-234-5656
- Cod Liver Oil, carlsonlabs.com, 1-888-234-5656
- L-Arginine Powder, carlsonlabs.com, 1-888 234-5656
- Vitamin K2 1 mg, Thorne, 1-800-228-1966
- Super K with K2, lef.com, 1-800-208-3444
- Peak K2 15 mg, y2khealthanddetox.com, 1-877-402-5450
- PhosChol, nutrasal.com, 1-800-364-4416
- Detoxamin, microzyme@mindpring.com, 1-877-656-4553
- DetoxMax Plus, bioimmune.com, 1-888-663-8844
- Detox Cocktail detailed in Chapter II
- Magnesium forms detailed in Chapter I
- Macrobiotic diet in Chapter V
- For interpretation of your blood work with myself via scheduled phone consultations, call 1-315-488-2846 for information.
- Folixor 1 mg sublingual, intensivenutrition.com
- NSC-24™ Beta Glucan Circulatory Formula, nsc24.com, 888-541-3997
- Nattokinase, Bio-Botanical, 800-775-4140
- Boluoke, Canada RNA, 866-287-8671
- Wobenzyme, Pain & Stress Center, 800-669-CALM
- Serrapeptase, Pain & Stress Center, 800-669-CALM
- IntraMin, druckerlabs.com, 1-972-881-2344

References:

Anand G, Life support. The big secret in health-care: rationing is here. With little guidance, workers on front lines decide who gets what treatment, *Wall Street Journal*, A1, A6, Sept.12, 2003

Kravitz RL, Bell RA, Thom DH, et al, Direct observation of request for clinical services in office practice. What do patients want and do they get it?, *Arch Intern Med*, 163: 1673-81, July 28, 2003

Sinatra ST, Sinatra J, *Lower Your Blood Pressure in Eight Weeks*, Ballantine Books, NY, 2003

Morales AJ, et al. Effects of replacement dose of dehydroepiandrosterone in men and women of advancing age, *J Clin Endocrinol Metab*, 78; 6:1360-67, June 1994

Barnhart Cate, et al, The effects of dehydroepiandrosterone supplementation on symptomatic peri-menopausal women and serum endocrine profiles, lipid parameters, and health-related quality of life, *J Clin Endocrinol Metab* 84; 11:3896-3902, Nov. 1999

Fogari R, Malacco E, Preti P, et al, Plasma testosterone in isolated systolic hypertension, *Hypertension* 42; 4, Oct. 2003

Kannel WB, Vasan RS, Levy D, Isolated relation of systolic blood pressure to risk of cardiovascular disease, *Hypertension* 42; 4:43-56, Oct. 2003

Muller M, et al., Endogenous sex hormones and cardiovascular disease in men, *J Clin Endocrinol Metab*, 88; 11: 5076-86, 2003

Cherrier MM, et al. Testosterone supplementation improves spatial and verbal memory in healthy older men, *Neurol*, 57; 1:80-88, July 10, 2001

Moffat SB, et al, Longitudinal assessment of serum free testosterone concentration predicts memory performance and cognitive status in elderly men, *J Clin Endocrinol Metab* 87; 11:5001-07, Nov 2002

Hak AE, et al, Low levels of endogenous androgens increase the risk of atherosclerosis in elderly men, *J Clin Endocrinol Metab* 87; 8:3632-39, Aug. 2002

Verghese J, et al, Low blood pressure and risk of dementia in very old individuals, *Neurol*, 61; 12: 1667-72, 2003

Verdecchia P, Schillaci G, Borgioni C, et al, Cigarette smoking, ambulatory blood pressure and cardiac hypertrophy in essential hypertension, *J Hypertension*, 13; 10:1209-15, Oct 13, 1995

Espeland MA, Whelton PK, Kostis JB, et al, Predictors and mediators of successful long-term withdrawal from antihypertensive medicines, *Arch Fam Med*, 8; 3:228-36, 1999

Langsjoen P, Willis R, Folkers K, Treatment of hypertension with coenzyme Q10, *Molec Aspects Med*, 15: suppl. S265-72, 1994

Digiesi V, Cantini E, Oradei A, Bisi G, Guarino GC, et al, Coenzyme Q10 in essential hypertension, *Molec Aspects Med* 1994;15(Supple):S257-72

Digiesi V, Cantini F, Brodbeck B, Effect of coenzyme Q10 on essential hypertension, *Curr Ther Res*, 47:841-5, 1990

Yamagami T, Iwamoto Y, Folkers K, Blomqvist CG, Reduction by coenzyme Q10 of hypertension induced by deoxycorticosterone and saline in rat, *Int J Vitam Nutr Res* 44:487-96, 1974

Garashi T, Nakajima Y, Tanaka M, Ohtake S, Effect of coenzyme Q10 on experimental hypertension in rats and dogs, *J Pharmacol Exp Ther* 189:149-56, 1974

Singh RB, Niaz MA, Rastogi SS, Shukla PK, Thakur AS, Effects of hydrosoluble coenzyme Q10 on blood pressure and insulin resistance in hypertensive patients with coronary artery disease, *J Hum Hypertens* 13; 3:203-8, Mar 1999

Burke BE, Neuenschwander R, Olson RD, Randomized, double-blind, placebo-controlled trial of coenzyme Q10 in isolated systolic hypertension, *South Med J*, 94; 11:1112-17, 2001

Fairfield K. M., Fletcher AH, Vitamins for chronic disease prevention in adults: Scientific review, *J Am Med Assoc*, 287; 23: 3116-3126, June 19, 2002

Fletcher RH, Fairfield K. M., Vitamins for chronic disease prevention in adults: Clinical applications. *J Am Med Assoc*, 287; 23: 3127-3129, June 19, 2002

Rossouw JE, Writing Group for the Women's Health Initiative Investigators, Risks and benefits of estrogen plus progestin in healthy post menopausal women: Principal results from the Women's Health Initiative Randomized Controlled Trial, *J Am Med Assoc*, 288; 3: 3 21-3 33, July 17, 2002

Ames BN, Elson-Schwab I, Silver EA. High-dose vitamin therapy stimulates the variant enzymes with decreased coenzyme binding affinity (increased Km): relevance to genetic disease and polymorphisms. *Am J Clin Nutr*, 75: 616-658, 2002

Hodis HN, Mack WJ, Azen SP, et al, Serial coronary angiographic evidence that antioxidants vitamin intake reduces progression of coronary artery atherosclerosis, *Journal American Medical Association*, 273; 23: 1849-54, June 21, 1995

Sahyoun NR, Jacques PF, Russell RM, Mayer J, Carotenoids, vitamins C and E, and mortality in an elderly population, *Am J Epidem*, 144; 5: 501-11, Sept. 1, 1996

Losonczy KG, Harris TB, Havlik RJ, Vitamin E and vitamin C supplement use and risk of all-cause and coronary heart disease mortality in older persons: the Established Populations for Epidemiologic Studies of the Elderly, *Am J Clin Nutr*, 64; 2:190-96, Aug. 1996

Hu FB, et al, Fish and Long-chain all mega- 3 fatty acid intake and risk of coronary heart disease and total mortality in diabetic women, *Circulation* 17; 14: 1852-57, April 15, 2003

Pelton R, et al, *Drug-Induced Nutrient Depletion Handbook*, (1-877-837-5394)

Seyama Y, et al, Comparative effects of vitamin K2 and vitamin E on experimental arterio-sclerosis, *Internat J Vit Nutr Res*, 69:23-26, 1999

Ronden JE, et al, Modulation of arterial thrombosis tendency in rats by vitamin K and its sidechains, *Atherosclerosis* 132:61-7, 1997

Jancin B, Vitamin K cuts heptocellular cancer mortality, *Fam Pract News*, 16, July 15, 2002

Houston MC, The role of vascular biology, nutrition and neutraceuticals in the prevention and treatment of hypertension, *J Am Nutraceut Assoc*, suppl. Apr. 2002

Shippen E, *The testosterone Syndrome*, M. Evans & Co., NY, 1998

Morales AJ, et al, Effects of replacement dose of dehydroepiandrosterone in men and women of advancing age, *J Clin Endocrinol Metab*, 78; 6:1360-67, June 1994

Barnhart C, et al, The effects of dehydroepiandrosterone supplementation to symptomatic menopausal women on serum endocrine profiles, lipid parameters, and health-related quality of life, *J Clin Endocrinol Metab* 84; 11:3896 -3902, Nov 1999

Fogari R, Malacco E, Preti P, et al, Plasma testosterone in isolated systolic hypertension, *Hypertension* 42; 4, Oct. 2003

Kannel WB, Vasan RS, Levy D, Is there a relation of systolic blood pressure to risk of car-diovascular disease and are there critical values?, *Hypertension* 42; 4: 43-56, Oct. 2003

Trivedi DP, et al, Effects of four monthly oral vitamin D3 (cholecalciferol) supplementation on fractures and mortality in men and women living in the community: randomized dou-ble-blind controlled trial, *Brit Med J*, 326; 7387: 469-63, Mar. 1, 2003

Thomas MK, Lloyd-Jones DM, Finkelstein JS, et al, Hypovitaminosis D in medical inpa-tients, *New Engl J Med*, 338; 12:777-83, 1998

LeBoff MS, Kohlmeier L, Glowacki J, et al, Occult vitamin D deficiency in postmenopausal U.S. women with acute hip fracture, *J Am Med Assoc*, 28; 281(16):1505-11, 1999

Vieth R, Vitamin D nutrition and its potential health benefits for bone, cancer and other conditions, *J Nutr Environ Med*, 11:275-91, 2001

Hanni LL, Huarfner LH, Ljunghall S, et al, Vitamin C is related to blood pressure and other cardiovascular risk factors in middle-aged man, Am J *Hypert*, 8: 894-901, 1995

Lind L, Wengle BO, Junghall S, Blood pressure is lowered by vitamin D (alphacalcidol) during long-term treatment of patients with intermittent hypercalcemia, *Acta Med Scand*, 222: 423-27, 1987

Lind L, Lithell H, Skarfos E, et al, Reduction of blood pressure by treatment with alphacal-cidol, *Acta Med Scand* 223: 211-17, 1988

Lind L, Wengle BO, Ljunghall S, et al, Hypertension in primary hyperparathyroidism—reduction of blood pressure by long-term treatment with vitamin D (alphacalcidol). A double blind, placebo-controlled study, *Am J Hypert*, 1: 397-402, 1988

Kurtz TW, Morris RC, Dietary intake of vitamin D as a determinant of deoxycorticosterone hypertension, *Hypert*, 8: 833 abstr., 1986

Chapuy M-C, Preziosi P, Meunier PJ, et al, Prevalence of vitamin D insufficiency in adult normal population, *Osteoporosis Internat*, 7: 439-43, 1997

Kitch BT, Vamvakas EC, Finkelstein JS, et al, Hypovitaminosis D in medical inpatients, *New Engl J Med*, 338: 777-83, 1998

Trivedi DP, Doll R, Khaw KT, Effect of four monthly oral vitamin D 3 (cholecalciferol) supplementation on fractures and mortality in men and women living in the community: randomized double-blind controlled trial, *Brit Med J*, 326: 4 69-74, 2003

Heaney RP, Dowell MS, Bendich A, et al, Calcium absorption varies within the reference range for serum 25-hydroxyvitamin D, *J Am Coll Nutr*, 22; 2: 142-46, 2003

Ravid A, Rocker D, Koren R, et al, 1,25-Dihydroxyvitamin D3 enhances the susceptibility of breast cancer cells to doxorubicin-induced oxidative damage. *Cancer Res* 59; 4:862-67, 1999

Vasquez A, Manso G, Cannell J, The clinical importance of vitamin D (cholecalciferol): a paradigm shift with implications for all health-care providers, *Altern Therap*, 10; 5:28-36, 2004

Zittermann A, Vitamin D in preventive medicine: are we ignoring the evidence? *Brit J Nutr*, 89:552-72, 2003

Yechiel E, Barenholz Y, Relationships between membrane lipid composition and biological properties of rat myocytes. Effects of aging and manipulation of lipid composition, *J Biol Chem*, 260; 16:9123-31, Aug. 5, 1985

Yechiel E, Henis YE, Barenholz Y, Aging of rat heart fibroblast: relationship between lipid composition, membrane organization and biological properties, *Biochim Biophys Acta*, 859; 1: 95-104, July 10, 1986

Yechiel E, Barenholz Y, Cultured heart cell reaggregates: a model for studying relationships between aging and lipid composition, *Biochim Biophys Acta*, 859; 1: 105-9, July 10, 1986

Bar LK, Barenholz Y, Thompson TE, Effect of sphingomyelin composition on the phase structure of phosphatidylcholine-sphingomyelin bilayers, *Biochem*, 3; 9: 2507-16, Mar. 4, 1997

Samochowiec L, On the action of the essential phospholipids in experimental atherosclerosis, page 211-26, in Peeters H,ed., *Phosphatidylcholine, Biochemical and Clinical Aspects of The Essential Phospholipids*, Springer-Verlag,, NY 1976

Howard AN, Patelski J, Effect of EPA on the lipid metabolism of the arterial wall and other tissues, page 187-200, in Peeters H,ed., *Phosphatidylcholine, Biochemical and Clinical Aspects of The Essential Phospholipids*, Springer-Verlag,, NY 1976

Samochowiec L, Kadlubowsha D, Rozewicka L, Investigations in experimental atherosclerosis: part 1: The effects of phosphatidylcholine (EPL) on experimental atherosclerosis in white rats, *Atherosclerosis* 23: 305-17, 1976

Samochowiec L, Kadlubowsha D, Rozewicka L, Kuzna W, Szyska K, Investigations in experimental atherosclerosis: part 2: The effects of phosphatidylcholine (EPL) on experimental atherosclerotic changes in miniature pigs, *Atherosclerosis* 23: 319-31 1976

Stafford W. W., Day CE, Regression of atherosclerosis affected by intravenous phospholipid, *Artery*, 1: 106-114, 1975

Gordon CM, et al, *Arch Ped Adolesc Med*, 158: 531-37, 2004

Pierpaoli W, Regelson W, Colman C, *The Melatonin Miracle*, Simon & Schuster, NY 1995

Altura BM, Altura BT, Interactions of Mg and K on blood vessels – aspects in view of hypertension. Review of present status and new findings. *Magnesium*, 3 (4-6); 175-194, 1984

Holick MF, Vitamin D: Importance in the prevention of cancer, type I diabetes, heart disease, and osteoporosis, *Am J Clin Nutr*, 79:362-71, 2004

Binkley N, Kruegar D, Drezner MK, et al, Assay variation confounds the diagnosis of hypovitaminosis D: A call for standardization, *J Clin Enodocrinol Metab*, 89; 7:3152-7, 2004

Liu J, Atamna H, Kuratsune, Ames BN, Delaying brain mitochondrial aging with mitochondrial antioxidant and metabolites, *Ann NY Acad Sci* 953:133-166, 2002

Fairfield KM, Fletcher RH, Levinson W, Vitamins for chronic disease prevention in adults: Scientific review, *J Am Med Assoc*, 287; 23: 3116-3126, Jun 19, 2002

Fletcher RH, Fairfield K. M, Levinson W, Vitamins for chronic disease prevention in adults: Clinical applications, *J Am Med Asso,c* 287; 23: 3127-29, Jun 19, 2002

Prasad KN, Cole WC, *Cancer and Nutrition*, IOS Press, Washington D.C., 1998

Moss RW, *Antioxidants Against Cancer*, Equinox Press, Brooklyn, 2000

Boushney CJ, et al, A quantitative assessment of plasma homocysteine as a risk factor for vascular disease, *J Amer Med Assoc*, 274:1049-57, 1995

Carson NAJ, et al, Homocysteinuria: a new inborn error of metabolism associated with mental deficiency, *Arch Dis Child*, 38:425-36, 1963

Rosenberg IH, Rosenberg LE, The implications of genetic diversity for nutrient requirements: The case of folate, *Nutr Rev*, 56; 2:s47-53, 1998

Farvid MS, Jalali M, Hosseini M, et al, The impact of vitamins and/or mineral supplementation on blood pressure in type 2 diabetes, *J Am Coll Nutr* 23; 3:272-79, 2004

Gaby AR, "Sub-laboratory" hypothyroidism and the empirical use of Armour® thyroid, *Alt Med Rev,* 9; 2:157-79, 2004

Barnes BO, Hypertension and the thyroid gland, *Clin Exp Pharmacol Physiol,* suppl 2:167-70, 1975

Menof P, Essential hypertension: its control by a new method. A preliminary report, *S Afr Med J,* 24:172-80, 1950

Dernellis J, et al, Effects of thyroid replacement therapy on arterial blood pressure in patients with hypertension and hypothyroidism, *Am Heart J,* 143:718-24, 2002

Hussein WI, it al, Normalization of hyperhomocysteinemia with L-thyroxine in hypothyroidism, *Ann Intern Med,* 131:348-51, 1999

Vrca VB, Skreb F, Cepelak I, et al, Supplementation with antioxidants in the treatment of Grave's disease: the effect on glutathione peroxidase activity and concentration of selenium, *Clin Chim Acta,* 3415-63, 2004

Jones K, Hughes K, MeKenna DJ, et al, Coenzyme Q-10 and cardiovascular health, *Integrative Med,* 3; 1:46-55, Feb/Mar 2004

Singh RB, Niaz MA, Rastogi SS, et al, Effect of hydrosoluble coenzyme Q10 on blood pressures and insulin resistance in hypertensive patients with coronary artery disease, *J Hum Hypertens,* 13:327-38, 1999

Boger RH, Borlak J, Bode-Boger SM, et al, LDL cholesterol upregulates synthesis of asymmetrical dimethylarginine in human endothelial cells: involvement of S-adenosylmethionine-dependent methyltransferases, *Circ Res* 87; 2:99-105, 2000

Orimo H, et al, Effects of mentetrenone on the bone and mineral metabolism in osteoporosis: a double-blind placebo-controlled trial, *J Bone Miner Metab,* 16; 2:106-12, 1998

Asakura H, et al, Vitamin K administration to elderly patients with osteoporosis induces no hemostatic activation, *Osteoporosis Int,* 12; 12:996-1000, 2001

Habu D, et al, Role of vitamin K2 in the development of hepatocellular carcinoma in women with viral cirrhosis of the liver, *J Am Med Assoc,* 292; 3:358-61, 2004

Cavallo A, et al, Blood pressure-lowering effect of melatonin in type 1 diabetes, *J Pineal Res,* 36; 4:262-66, May 2004

Lahiri DK, et al, Dietary supplementation with melatonin reduces levels of amyloid beta-peptides in the murine cerebral cortex, , *J Pineal Res,* 36; 4: 2 24-31, May 2004

Sener G, et al, Melatonin reverses urinary system and aortic damage in the rat due to chronic nicotine administration, *J Pharm Pharmacol,* 56; 3:359-66, March 2004

Tan DX, et al, Melatonin: a hormone, a tissue factor, and autocoid, a paracoid, and antioxidant vitamin, *J Pineal Res*, 34; 1:75-78, Jan. 2003

Zhang YC, et al, Melatonin attenuates beta-amyloid-induced inhibition of neurofilament expression, *Acta Pharmacol Sin*, 25; 4: 4 47-51, Apr. 2004

Kalea AZ, Harris PD, Klimis-Zacas DJ, Dietary manganese suppresses *a*1 adrenergic receptor-mediated vascular contraction, *J Nutr Biochem*, 16:44-49, 2005

Goldhaber SZ, American Public Health Association, Deep-vein thrombosis: Advancing awareness to protect patients lives, White Paper: *Public Health Leadership Conference on Deep-Vein Thrombosis*, Washington D.C., Feb. 26, 2003

daRocha M, Silva, DeFilippe, et al, Infection prevention in patients with severe multiple trauma with the immunomodulators beta 1-3 polyglucose (glucan), *Surg Gynecol Obstet*, 177: 383-88, 1993

Ohno N, et al, Effect of beta-glucans on the nitric oxide synthesis by peritoneal macrophages in mice, *Biol Pharmacol Bull*, 19:608-12, 1996

Jordan BF, Gregoire V, Demeure RJ, Gallez B, et al, Insulin increases the sensitivity of tumors to irradiation: involvement of an increase in tumor oxygenation mediated by a nitric oxide-dependent decrease of the tumor cells oxygen consumption, *Cancer Res*, 15; 16 (12): 3555-61, June 2002

Braga PC, et al, Effects of Serrapeptase on muco-ciliary clearance in patients with chronic bronchitis, *Curr Ther Res*, 29;5:738-44, 1981

Carratu L, et al, Physio-chemical and rheological research on mucolytic activity of Serrapeptase in chronic broncho-pneumopathies, *Curr Ther Res*, 28; 6:930 7-51, 1980

Mazzonie A, et al, Evaluation of of Serrapeptase in acute or chronic inflammation of oto-rhinolaryngology pathology: a multicenter, double-blind randomized trial versus placebo, J *Int Med Res*, 18; 5:370 9-88, 1990

Batkin S, et al, Antimetastatic effect of bromelain, *J Cancer Res Clin Oncol*, 114:507-8, 1988

Batkin S, et al, Modulation of pulmonary metastasis (Lewis lung carcinoma) by bromelain, an extract of the pineapple stem (Ananas comosus), *Cancer Invest*, 6:421-2, 1988

Wang R, et al, Effects of Fleroxacin combined with urokinase or earthworm kinases on bacterial biofilms, *Acta Pharmaceut Sinica*, 9; 34: 662-65, 1995

Sumi H, Hamada H, Tsushima H, Mihara H, Muraki H, A novel fibrinolytic enzyme, nattokinase, in the vegetable cheese natto: A typical and popular soybean food in the Japanese diet. *Experimentia* 43; 10: 1110-11, 1987

Sumi H, Hamada H, Nakanishi K, Hirantani H. Enhancement of the fibrinolytic activity in plasma by oral administration of nattokinase. *Acta Haematol* 84: 139-143, 1990

Ohkura I, Komatsuzaki T, et al. The level of serum lysozyme activity in animals fed a diet containing natto bacilli (Japanese), *Med Bio* 102:335-337, 1981

Fujita M, Hong K, Ito Y, Fujii R, Kariya K, Nishimuro S. Thrombolytic effect of nattokinase on a chemically induced thrombosis model in rats. *Biol Pharm Bull* 18;10:1387-1391, 1995

Fujita M, Hong K, Ito Y, Misawa S, Takeuchi N, Kariya K, Nishimuro S. Transport of nattokinase across the rat intestinal tract. *Biol Pharm Bull* 18;9:1194-11 96, 1995

Okamoto A, Hanagata H, Kawamura Y, Yanagida F. Anti-hypertensive substances in fermented soybean, natto. *Plants Foods Human Nutrition* 47; 1: 39-47, 1995

Chapter VII

The Mind and Soul Connection

There's no question that your mind controls your body physiology. Without touching you, without injecting you, without getting near you, I can make your heart race, your blood pressure soar, boost your breathing rate, facial flushing, and much more within seconds by just delivering horrible news. I know a woman who had a stroke within seconds of hearing of her husband's death, and we have all heard of heart attacks, elevated blood pressure or arrhythmias leading to strokes within seconds of devastating news. The power of the mind to send out regulatory hormones and cytokines can be more powerful than any drugs.

This awesome power of the mind over your health extends to your day to day moods. In one study from the Mayo Clinic people who were pessimistic had a 19% increase in early death over optimists (*Murata*). And, you guessed it, an excess of chronic stress pours out inflammatory mediators that damage the walls of arteries and blood vessels causing Mr. ED (*Black*). Repressed anger and hostility likewise can raise your homocysteine levels and lead to Mr. ED (endothelial dysfunction), vasculitis, hypertension, organ death, or what ever label you want to give it (*Stoney*). Gosh, you've gotten smart! Clearly stress raises homocysteine levels and leads to endothelial dysfunction/hypertension and early death. Dr. Steven Sinatra, a well-respected New England cardiologist and author of a great book on hypertension has published papers showing that blood vessels can burst with suppressed anger and emotional stress (*Sinatra*).

Studies have also shown the power of prayer, and the power of positive relaxed feelings that benefit folks regardless of whether they have cancer, heart disease or any other disease (*Hiilakivi-Clarke, Byrd, Denollet*). I believe these health-controlling emotions have the best chance of stemming from a firm belief system rooted in proof.

Since life is full of constant stressors, we need a rescue that transcends far beyond the day-to-day hassles we all face. Having scoured the literature of psychiatry, psychology, molecular biochemistry, and environmental medicine it appears to me that there's only one solution that can make a major difference in one's chronic stress level. And that in my opinion can only come from an understanding of a much more encompassing view of our purpose that dwarfs our earthly struggles. By diminishing their significance in relation to what is really important, it provides a steadying focus. It becomes our foundation.

Boosting Spirituality is Healthful for the Immune System

A mounting body of evidence shows that family time spent together, as well as nurturing a belief system in a supreme being, not only improves ethics, morals and compassionate social skills in children, but is nurturing for the *neuropsychoimmunology* of the body, the brain-body-hormone connection. **In short, a healthy spirituality boosts the immune system** (*Larson*). That's one reason I'm excited about a few of the over hundred books I have read this year that I can't hold myself back from telling you about. One of my interests is apologetics (the study of the evidence for Christ's birth, life, resurrection and being God incarnate). Besides the many books that provide this evidence that I showed you in (the last chapter of) *Depression Cured At Last!*, I've found many new (to me) ones.

Why would I be interested in reading a book by the investigative reporter who discovered the inter-office memo proving that the Ford Motor Company knew its Pinto could burst into flames when hit from behind at only 20 mph, (which it did, killing innocent teenagers and others)? Why would I want to read a book by this same award-winning journalist and former legal editor of *The Chicago Tribune*, with a degree from Yale Law School who cracked crime cases that had stumped the police? Because this legal bulldog then went after the most important question in the world. Lee Strobel went far beyond Larry King who said of all the people in history, he would most like to interview Jesus Christ.

Strobel, a former agnostic legal investigative reporter par excellence didn't wait for Christ's PR agent to schedule a TV interview. He tackled the most important question in the world by tracking down the facts and sifting through the evidence using his legal/award-winning investigative reporter skills via interviews with top world authorities. As a consequence, he became a Christian after being assigned to interview 13 leading experts on the historical evidence for Jesus Christ. He documents this in his book, *The Case for Christ*. He then went on to write a second book interviewing even more experts, from theologians and historians to physicists, biologists, judges, law professors, and more in *The Case for Faith*. A next must-read is *The Case for a Creator*.

A former Hindu, Ravi Zacharias, who likewise interviewed leading world experts on the evidence for Christ, wrote another book that was equally convincing for me. He then proceeded to successfully present his evidence in spirited debates at Harvard, Oxford and other prestigious learning centers of the world. His book *Can Man Live Without God?* details this (all these books are available from 1-800-CHRISTIAN). If you need "convincing", these books should do it, and still many others are listed in Chapter 7 of *Depression Cured At Last!* (1-800-846-6687or prestigepublishing.com) as well as ongoing issues of *Total Wellness*.

I know that my friends, relatives, and colleagues who are Hindus, Jews, Muslims, Buddhists, agnostics or share other belief systems will not be offended. For those who know me, know that I use Christianity as an example of the power of spirituality in general, with my examples coming from Christianity, because that's the one that I'm personally most familiar with and convinced by. The bottom line is that spirituality has proven to be healthful in a multitude of ways, and what better time to take stock of your spiritual needs? Furthermore we need to protect ourselves against loss of religious freedom (*Robertson*).

Healing the Impossible Begins with God's Food

As I continually search for the molecular/biochemical evidence that enables folks to heal the impossible, I'm eternally and humbly reminded of many facts. For example, as I have documented in past *TW* newsletters, Harvard researchers have proven that high doses of beta-carotene actually cause the p53 cancer gene to revert back to a normal gene. In other words, after everything that high-tech medicine has to offer has failed, and folks were on their deathbeds, nutrients in god-designed foods were able to accomplish gene therapy which no expensive high tech scientist or genetic engineering company is capable of. What an incredibly clever molecular biochemical system has been designed in our bodies to dovetail with the healing provisions in food! That's one of the many reasons why the protocol in *the Wellness Against All Odds* book includes hourly carrot juicing as part of a program proven to more than quadruple cancer survival (references in 1999-2005 *TW*). When biochemists have broken down foods to determine their preventive and curative properties, they have discovered thousands of compounds designed to heal. Although medical libraries are full of the healing properties of foods, there is no money in it, in comparison to the sustained profits of the pharmaceutical and fast food manufacturers. And besides, it cures.

"Has not God made foolish the wisdom of the world?" (*I Cor: 1*), for example, by reversing or reprogramming the p53 cancer gene. You learned in Chapter V that a mere 4 stalks of celery are enough for some folks to reverse their hypertension. Food as a cure seems so simple, that it is easy to ridicule, especially if you want folks dependent on a lifetime of highly profitable drugs.

Columbia University researchers have shown that *95% of disease*, whether cancer, heart or any other disease *is caused by only two things: diet and environment* (references in *DOD*). And *Revelations* warns us that the polluters will pay. We need only recall from *Corinthians I* that the body is the temple of the Lord and if we defile it (fill it full of junk food, trans fatty acids, Olestra, etc.), God will punish us. Is it ironic that **sin and death began with cheating on the diet**, and even though we have free will, we still keep doing it? And why as believers are we called the "salt of the earth"? Salt preserves, keeps food from going bad, or rancid from bacterial destruction. Are we also supposed to protect the earth from man's defiling of it, as well as protect ourselves?

On Higher Ground

As I see it, the surest way to avoid the tsunamis of life is to be on higher ground. To be on a plane that dwarfs our earthly concerns by enabling us to focus on a much bigger picture. This can be accomplished in one word. And speaking of that word, it is the one word that when spoken can divide a room full of folks. It will create an immediate pause, as folks align themselves with those who support their views, and distance themselves from those who do not. No, it is not the name of a president, national figure, or political party, not the name of a terrorist. It is Jesus.

There is no question that He lived on this earth. That is an established historical fact, which no authorities from any discipline have evidence to refute. So, as C. S. Lewis has said, then the question boils down to was He or was He not the Son of God as He claimed to be? If he was not, he must be a lunatic, schizophrenic and a raving maniac to make such outrageous claims. But there was not one tiny shred of evidence that He was unstable or mentally incompetent.

Furthermore, there is voluminous evidence of His miracles, personality, birth, life, teachings, death and resurrection. Most historical facts come to press so long after the event that there are usually no longer any living witnesses to refute the claims. Not so with Jesus (*Strobel*). The descriptions, for example of the post-resurrection sightings of Jesus by hundreds of people were written within a decade or so, when most of the people were still alive and able to refute.

And many different people wrote them. Furthermore, many of the unique details of His life were forecasted and documented over 500 years in advance of His birth (*Isaiah*).

Because man has free will, and his faith hinges on that free will, it is up to him to investigate the most important question in his life. Jesus could have come as a wealthy czar or ruler, a highly visible political figure or revered philosopher. Instead He came as a humble human carpenter. He could have chosen His disciples from among the most prominent religious leaders, rabbis, priests or Pharisees, judges, orators, or statesmen of the day. But no, He chose 12 humble, mediocre humans, fishermen, a tax collector, political adversaries, nonbelievers, and even the one that was planned to mediate His death. Instead "He assembled a ragtag bunch of folks with unimpressive resumés" (*MacArthur*).

He could have had His resurrection first witnessed by prominent legal authorities, but no, He chose women, a class that was not even allowed to speak in court in those days. For "God has chosen the foolish things of the world to put to shame the wise, and God has chosen the weak things of the world to put to shame the things which are mighty;" (*I Corinthians* 27-29).

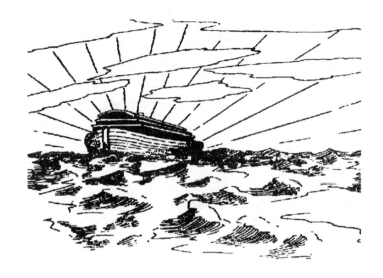

> *Are you ready to heal the impossible? Is anything impossible? You think we physicians are gods and that you could never do more for your health than we could? Remember that amateurs built the Ark, while professionals built the Titanic. The Ark is frozen intact in a glacier high on a treeless Turkish mountain, Mt. Ararat (Bright, Montgomery, LaHaye). The Titanic is disintegrating in the bottom of the ocean.*

If you think I am overwhelmed with the evidence for nutritional/environmental medicine, where we find the cause and cure for symptoms instead of drugging them to foster new diseases, you should see even a smattering of the evidence for the resurrection (*Stroble, Geisler, Stott, Craig, Habermas, Geivett, France, Bloomberg, Muncaster, Morison, Kreeft, etc*).

Or on a more personal level, I have only to reflect on some of the enormous blessings that I as one individual have received. In *Ephesians* it clearly states that God has a *preordained* purpose for us: "For we are God's workmanship,

241

created...to do good works, which God **prepared in advance for us to do"** (*Ephesians* 2:10). I can't deny the reality of that. I was the oldest of eight children, from a poor family. I was the first person on either side of the family to graduate from high school. With absolutely no money, I went to four years of college, then even more miraculously four years of medical school as a young woman in the early 1960s when women were not exuberantly welcomed to medical schools. What are the chances of that? To top it off, He gave me the most perfectly luscious husband in the universe who has nurtured, protected, guided and loved me more than my wildest dreams for 36 years. This has enabled us to quietly help enormous numbers of folks learn that they have the power within themselves to heal the impossible. And Luscious grows more luscious every day.

Or look at the years I suffered over 20 different "incurable" maladies. If I had been relieved of them, as I had prayed, it would have been a waste. Instead I was lead to find the causes and cures, which enabled me to teach others to do the same. Then in my continued searches for the evidence and scientific backup for every bit of this, it was sometimes literally dropped in my lap. I'm convinced God provided all this, through His miraculous design of the universe and everything in it. We all have a purpose. Discover yours.

If you had lived in 33 AD, what would you have put your money on for surviving into this century: the all-powerful Roman Empire or a group of poor people worshipping a crucified Jewish carpenter? And yet today the Roman Empire and its language are history, as even our coins and calendar reflect Christ. We name our kids Peter, Paul, John and James, and our dogs Caesar and Nero.

If you take a quick look around, you'll see we are surrounded by God's miraculous creations. Have you, like me, been suckered into the scheme presented in high school and college that the earth resulted from some big bang, and then we miraculously evolved from our ape uncles? You would do well to read the incontrovertible evidence from scholars around the world in divergent fields of how we could not possibly have life on this earth if one minute celestial parameter were changed (Strobel, *A Case For Creation*, 1-800-CHRISTIAN). The chance that all the correct physical attributes of the universe to sustain life on earth would be fulfilled by chance literally contains more zeros than we can fit on this page. Or take the chance that all the amazingly harmonious chemistry of the body "just happened". No, the evidence is overwhelming that there is a design that far exceeds human intelligence that purposely put us here (*Strobel, Meyer, Moreland, Witham, Behe, Carlson, Witham*). When you learn how exceedingly clever the whole universe is, right down to my main interest, the chemistry of healing the impossible, this is all a plan to provide us with the fun of endless, joyous discovery. But there is much more beyond that plan, and it extends right down to you and me.

In essence, here is the most important decision you will ever make in your life and the results extend far beyond this earthly life. As well, it gives birth to a peace and purpose that dwarfs our earthly struggles. So you might want to consider all of the evidence even more diligently than you assessed the evidence here for reversing your high blood pressure. For now, you have seen a minute amount of the evidence of how big business wants to a keep you sick forever (even calling it chronic illness), even though it is well known how to heal the impossible. Other forces are likewise

at work to keep you spiritually impoverished and unem
powered (*Gurnall, Eph 4-6, Rev 12, 20*).

The Total Load

Don't be scared off by all of the options I've given you. The
solution can be exceedingly simple. But since I'm addressing such a wide spectrum of individuals, I must make sure
you understand the total load. For the total package of
overload in your body determines how much you must do
in order to unload your system sufficiently, to enable your
body to heal itself. I don't know how sick you are or how
much you have abused your body. So let's look at other
options beyond the scope of this tome.

For starters, if the gut isn't healthy, you'll be indefinitely
stalled for complete healing. This is because the gut houses
over half the immune system and over half of the detoxification system, both crucial to healing the vascular tree. If
what I've written here is not sufficient to heal your gut, refer to *No More Heartburn*, which gives much more detail for
the entire gastrointestinal system.

Likewise if you are knocking yourself out to get rid of har-
bored chemicals, but you have a contaminated environment
that is tanking you up faster than you can get rid of them,
you can indefinitely stall success. *The E. I. Syndrome, Tired
or Toxic?*, and *Chemical Sensitivity* will guide you. And if
you have a serious disease like cancer, there is so much
more you need to know and do. I would suggest starting
with *Wellness Against All Odds*, then progressing to *You Are
What You Ate*, followed by *The Cure is in the Kitchen* and
Macro Mellow. If you have chronic pain of any sort, *Pain*

Free In 6 Weeks may provide a startlingly easy cure (plus the 2005 *Total Wellness*, as examples).

Depression Cured At Last! describes the total load of environmental, nutritional, and metabolic triggers for all diseases, using depression as an example. For it is not only the blueprint for beginning to figure out the causes and cures for every brain disorder, from migraines or ADD to seizures or schizophrenia, but for all disease. *The Scientific Basis for Selected Environmental Medicine Techniques* provides even more information, especially for physicians.

More importantly, there are critically important modalities that neither I nor anyone else has yet to write about that may be necessary for turning back the hands of time for you. For those who stay tuned to the monthly referenced newsletter, *Total Wellness,* they will find a multitude of exciting answers. I can't wait to tell you about them! I can't research and write fast enough! And they are designed to save you much money and side effects by learning how to heal and not need drugs. In the meantime, I do have personal scheduled phone consultations for folks who are not my patients, but cannot wait and would like to brainstorm personally with me about their options.

And last, but never least, as it says in the *Bible,* "Neither do men pour new wine into old wineskins" (*Mt* 9:17). You need a clean body, free of its lifetime of stored chemicals. *Detoxify or Die* shows you how to clean it in detail. And what good is it to have a clean, detoxified body but a trashed, toxic soul? As an integral part of the total load, there is a huge reservoir of information substantiating how not only pivotal the mental attitude and psyche are, but our individual belief system is for healing. I have seen folks heal the impossible after detoxing their souls. Have you explored all the evidence you need to make the most important decision of your life?

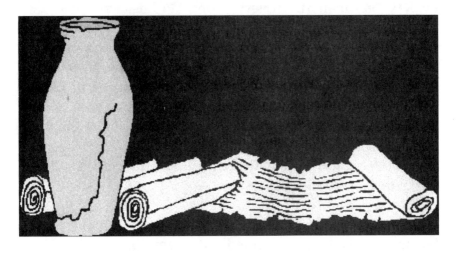

"Neither do men pour new wine into old wineskins" (Mt 9:17). What good is it to have a clean body but a trashed soul?

On the flip side, I've seen the opposite phenomenon in over 35 years of medical practice. Folks burdened with anger, guilt, hatred, jealousy, hurt, shame, and other health-robbing emotions are indefinitely stalled for healing, until they can rise above and forgive. Genuine forgiveness appears to be critical for dissolving **damaging emotions that can retard healing indefinitely.** Remember that foremost, "a cheerful heart is good medicine" (*Proverbs* 17: 22). "Forgive, and you will be forgiven. Give, and it will be given to you. A good measure, pressed down, shaken together and running over, will be poured into your lap. For with the measure you use, it will be measured to you." (*Luke* 6: 38)

For me personally, *The Holy Bible* (King James Version) has been a literal and figurative Godsend. If it makes no sense and the reading is difficult, start with my favorite book that I have read over seven times, *Adventuring Through the Bible*, by Ray Stedman (Discovery House Publishers, 1-800-653-8333). Or to explain the Biblical miracles and mysteries, *The Scientific Approach to Christianity* and *The Scientific Approach to Biblical Mysteries* (New Leaf Press, PO Box 311, Green Forest AR 72638). A former agnostic rocket scientist, Robert Faid, who was miraculously healed of his cancer, wrote them. He had decided to scientifically investigate whether there was anything to this Christianity that his wife professed healed him. He ended up being fully converted and wrote these great books.

It may appear to the uninitiated that I am merely out to sell books. The fact is I was gifted with over 20 incurable diagnoses, all of which are healed. I have devoted my life to trying to figure out the causes and cures for disease, and then how to empower folks like you with that knowledge. I could easily be retired now, but my goal is to progressively bring this knowledge to a level where even more precious people can benefit. For each of us must "use whatever gift he has received to serve others," (*I Peter* 4:10).

In an era out of control, ruled by ironclad forces with unhealthy agendas, I have no unrealistic goal of fame or fortune, but am intent upon providing the life-saving information I have learned to help others who are ready to use it. I believe in the old adage, that when the student is ready, the teacher appears. And "Seek and you will find" (*Matt.* 7: 7).

I hope this abbreviated tome gives you a small appreciation for the magnificence of the natural, God-given healing capability that has been programmed in you. I hope it has instilled in you an appreciation for the awesome power you have over your health. For each day you are silently called upon to exercise decisions that will lead to your getting either healthier or not. The tough part is you are surrounded by medical "authorities" who fail to comprehend the power you have. Their major solution for your every symptom is a drug.

Above all, remember that the more one studies molecular biochemistry, the more convinced he must be of the presence of a Master Biochemist who has absolutely and miraculously designed the human body to heal, against all odds (*Strobel*). And nutrients in our foods are orchestrated to harmonize and heal the body. In that case, shouldn't you make it a top priority to know more about this Master Biochemist?

In closing, remember from the Bible how Eve was duped by the serpent to disobey God's commands? He gave bad advice.

"Now the serpent was more crafty than any of the wild animals the Lord God had made. He said to the woman, "Did God really say, 'You must not eat from any tree in the garden? '" (Genesis 3: 1).

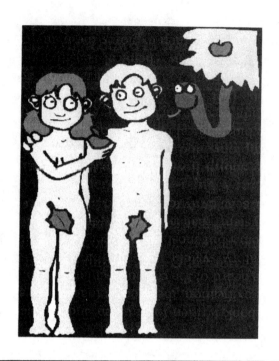

Later that day, "the Lord God said to the woman,' What is this you have done?'"

"The woman said, 'The serpent deceived me, and I ate.'" (Genesis 3: 13).

Isn't it a coincidence that the caduceus symbol for medicine is a winged staff with two serpents entwined?

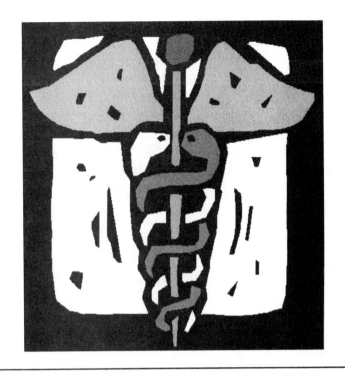

The serpent is still deceiving us.

Sources:

If you would like some places where your doctor (and you) could learn more about this type of medicine, have him contact:

- The Institute for Functional Medicine
  for physician symposia, courses, books, tapes
  functionalmedicine.org, 1-800-228-0622, fax 1-253-853-6766
- The American Environmental Health Foundation
  for physician symposia, books, less toxic products
  Aehf.com or 1-800-428-2343
- *Total Wellness* monthly subscription newsletter by this author, public lectures, books, radio, TV, physician lectures, personal non-patient phone consultations and laboratory interpretations prestigepublishing.com or 1-800-846-6687

References:

Black PH, Garbutt LD, Stress, inflammation and cardiovascular disease, *J Psychosom Res*, 52:1-23, Jan. 2002

Stoney CM, Engebretson TO, Plasma homocysteine concentrations are positively associated with hostility and anger, *Life Sci*, 66: 2267-75, 2000

Sinatra ST, *Heartbreak and Heart Disease*, Keats Publishing, New Canaan CT, 1998

Murata TC, Colligan RC, Offord KP, et al, Optimist vs. pessimists: Survival rate among medical patients over 30-year period, *Mayo Clin Proc*, 75: 141-43, 2000

Hiilakivi-Clarke L, et al, Psychosocial factors in the development and progression of breast cancer: a review. *Breast Cancer Res Treat*, 29: 141-60, 1993

Byrd RC, Positive therapeutic effects of intercessory prayer in a coronary care unit population, *South Med J*, 81: 826-29, 1988

Denollet J, et al, Personality as independent predictor of long-term mortality in patients with coronary heart disease, *Lancet*, 347: 414-21, 1996

Brett AS, Jersild P, "Inappropriate" treatment near the end of life. Conflict between religious convictions and clinical judgment, *Arch Intern Med* , 163: 1645-49, July 28, 2003

Sinatra ST, Chawla S, Aortic dissection associated with anger, suppressed rage, and acute emotional stress, *J Cardiopulm Rehab*, 6:197-99, 1986

Ames BN, Elson-Schwab I, Silver EA. High-dose vitamin therapy stimulates the variant enzymes with decreased coenzyme binding affinity (increased Km): relevance to genetic disease and polymorphisms. *Am J Clin Nutr, 75*: 616-658, 2002

Hodis HN, Mack WJ, Azen SP, et al, Serial coronary angiographic evidence that antioxidants vitamin intake reduces progression of coronary artery atherosclerosis, *Journal American Medical Association*, 273; 23: 1849-54, June 21, 1995

Sahyoun NR, Jacques PF, Russell RM, Mayer J, Carotenoids, vitamins C and E, and mortality in an elderly population, *Am J Epidem*, 144; 5: 501-11, Sept. 1, 1996

Losonczy KG, Harris TB, Havlik RJ, Vitamin E and vitamin C supplement use and risk of all-cause and coronary heart disease mortality in older persons: the Established Populations for Epidemiologic Studies of the Elderly, *Am J Clin Nutr*, 64; 2:190-96, Aug. 1996

Hu FB, et al, Fish and Long-chain all mega-3 fatty acid intake and risk of coronary heart disease and totaled mortality in diabetic women, *Circulation* 17; 14:1852-57, April 15, 2003

MacArthur J., *Twelve Ordinary Men*, W Publishing, Thomas Nelson, Nashville TN, 2002

Montgomery JW, *The Quest for Noah's Ark*, Bethany Fellowship, Minn. MN, 1974

La Haye T, Morris J, *The Ark On Ararat*, Thomas Nelson Publ, NY, 1974

Bright RC, *The Ark, A Reality?*, Ranger Assoc, NY, 1989

Ogilvie LJ Chaplain of the U.S. Senate, *One Quiet Moment*, Harvest House Publ., Eugene OR, 1997

Ogilvie LJ Chaplain of the U.S. Senate, *Conversations With God*, Harvest House Publ., Eugene OR, 1993

Geisler N, Howe T, *When Critics Ask*, Victor Books, Wheaton IL, 1992

Geisler NL, *A Popular Survey of the Old Testament*, Baker Books, Grand Rapids MI, 2003

Strobel, L, *The Case For Christ*, Zondervan, Grand Rapid MI, (1-800-CHRISTIAN), 1998

Strobel, L, *The Case For a Creator*, Zondervan, Grand Rapid MI, (1-800-CHRISTIAN), 2004

Geisler N L, *Christian Apologetics*, Prince Press, Peabody MA, (1-800-CHRISTIAN), 2003

Stott JRW, Basic Christianity, Wm. B. Eerdmans Publ., Grand Rapid MI, (also 1-800-CHRISTIAN), 1971

Strobel, L, *The Case For Faith*, Zondervan, Grand Rapid MI, (1-800-CHRISTIAN), 2000

Bloomberg C, *The Historical Reliability of the Gospels*, Downers Grove IL, InterVarsity Press, 1987

Bruce FF, *The New Testament Documents: Are they reliable?*, Eerdmans, Grand Rapis, MI, 1960

France RT, *The Evidence for Jesus*, Downers Grove IL, InterVarsity Press, 1986

Bloomberg C, The historical reliability of the New Testament", in *Reasonable Faith* by Wm Lane Craig, 193-231, Westchester IL, Crossway, 1994

Bruce FF, *Jesus and Christian Origins Outside the New Testament*, Downers Grove IL, Inter-Varsity Press, 1974

Habermas G, *The Historical Jesus*, College Press, Joplin MO, 1996

Habermas G, Licona M, *The Case for the Resurrection*, 1-800-CHRISTIAN

Muncater RO, *Evidence for Jesus*, 1-800-CHRISTIAN

Kreeft P, Tacelli RK, *Handbook of Christian Apologetics*, 1-800-CHRISTIAN

McDowell J, Wilson B, *He Walked Among Us*, Nelson, Nashville TN, 1994

Geisler NL, *Christian Apologetics*, 1-800-CHRISTIAN

Finegan J, *The Archaeology of the New Testament*, Princeton, Princeton Univ Press, 1992

Boyd GA, *Cynic Sage or Son of God?*, BridgePoint, Wheaton IL, 1995

Craig WL, Did Jesus rise from the dead?, in Wilkins MJ, Moreland JP, eds., *Jesus Under Fire*, 147-82, Grand Rapids, Zondervan, 1995

Craig WL, *Knowing the Truth About the Resurrection*, Servant, Ann Arbor MI, 1988

Craig WL, The empty tomb of Jesus, *In Defense of Miracles*, Geivett RD and Habermans GR, eds., 247-61, Downers Grove IL, InterVarsity Press, 1997

Edwards WD, et al, On the physical death of Jesus Christ, *J Amer Med Assoc*, 1455-63, Mar 21, 1986

Foreman D, *Crucify Him*, Grand Rapids, Zondervan 1990

Ankerberg J, Weldon J, *Ready With an Answer*, Eugene OR, Harvest House, 1997

Habermas G, Flew A, *Did Jesus Rise From the Dead? The Resurrection Debate*, Harper & Row, San Francisco, 1987

Morison F, *Who Moved the Stone?* Grand Rapids, Zondervan, 1987

Craig WL, *The Son Rises: Historical Evidence for the Resurrection of Jesus*, Chicago, Moody Press, 1981

Meyer SC, Evidence for design in physics and biology, in *Science and Evidence for Design in the Universe*, Behe MJ, Dembski WA, Meyer SC, eds., Ignatius, San Francisco, 1999

Carlson RF, ed., *Science and Christianity: Four Views*, InterVarsity, Downer's Grove IL, 2000

Moreland JP, *Christianity and the Nature of Science*, Grand Rapids MI, Baker, 1989

Witham L, *By Design: Science and the Search for God*, Encounter, San Francisco, 2003

Moreland JP, Nielsen K, *Does God Exist?*, Amherst NY, Prometheus, 1993

Robertson P, *Courting Disaster: How the Supreme Court is Usurping the Power of Congress and the People*, 1-800-CHRISTIAN

Stedman R, *Adventuring Through the Bible*, Discovery House Publishers, 1-800-653-8333

Faid RW, *The Scientific Approach to Christianity*, New Leaf Press, PO Box 311, Green Forest AR 72638

Faid RW, *The Scientific Approach to Biblical Mysteries*, New Leaf Press, PO Box 311, Green Forest AR 72638

Larson DB, Larson SS, *The Forgotten Factor in Physical and Mental Health: What Does the Research Show?*, National Institute for Healthcare Research, 211 Wilson Blvd, Ste. 1130, Arlington VA 22201, 703-527-NIHR,1992

Sinatra ST, Sinatra J, *Lower Your Blood Pressure in Eight Weeks*, Ballentine Books, NY, 2003

Strobel L, *The Case for Easter*, 1-888-7000-CRI

Strobel L, *God's Outrageous Claims*, 1-800-CHRISTIAN

Craig WL, *Reasonable Faith: Christian Truth and Apologetics*, 1-888-7000-CRI

Ceisler NL, *Why I Am a Christian*, 1-888-7000-CRI

Geisler NL, *When Critics Ask*, 1-888-7000-CRI

Chapin A, *365 Bible Promises for People Who Worry*, tyndale.com

Gurnall W, *The Christian in Complete Armour*, Moody Press, Chicago

Geisler NL, *A Popular Survey of the Old Testament*, Baker Books, Grand Rapids, 1-800-CHRISTIAN or christianbook.com

MacArthur J, *Hard to Believe*, Thomas Nelson Publ., Nashville

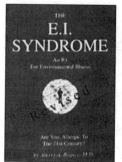

The E.I. Syndrome, Revised is a 635 page book that is necessary for people with **environmental illness**. It explains chemical, food, mold, and Candida sensitivities, nutritional deficiencies, testing methods and how to do the various environmental controls and diets in order to get well.

Many docs buy this by the hundreds and make them mandatory reading for patients, as it contains many pearls about getting well that are not found anywhere else. In this way it increases the fun of practicing medicine, because patients are on a higher educational level and office time is more productive for more sophisticated levels of wellness. It covers hundreds of facts that make the difference between E.I. victims versus E.I. conquerors. It helps patients become active partners in their care and thereby get better results, while avoiding doctor burnout. It covers the gamut of the diagnosis and treatment of environmentally induced symptoms.

Because the physician author was a severe universal reactor who has recovered, this book contains mountains of clues to wellness. As a result, many have written that they healed themselves of resistant illnesses of all types by reading this book. This is in spite of the fact that no consulted physicians were able to diagnose or effectively treat them. If you are not sure what causes your symptoms, this is a great start.

Many veteran sufferers have written that they had read many books on aspects of allergy, chronic Candidiasis and chemical sensitivity and thought that they knew it all. Yet (they wrote that) what they learned *in* **The E.I. Syndrome, Revised** enabled them to reach that last pinnacle of wellness.

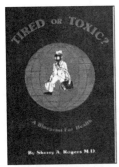 *Tired or Toxic?* is a 400 page book, and the first book that describes the mechanism, diagnosis and treatment of chemical sensitivity, complete with scientific references. It is written for the layman and physician alike and explains the many vitamin, mineral, essential fatty acid and amino acid analyses that help people detoxify everyday chemicals more efficiently and hence get rid of baffling symptoms, including chronic pain.

It is the first book written for laymen and physicians to describe xenobiotic detoxification, the process that allows all healing to occur. You have heard of the cardiovascular system, you have heard of the respiratory system, the gastrointestinal system, and the immune system. But most have never heard of the chemical detoxification system, that is the main determinant of whether we have chemical sensitivity, cancer, and in fact every disease.

This program shows how to diagnose and treat many resistant everyday symptoms and use molecular medicine techniques. It also gives the biochemical mechanisms in easily understood form, of how Candida creates such a diversity of symptoms and how the macrobiotic diet heals "incurable" end stage metastatic cancers. It is a great book for the physician you are trying to win over, and shows you how chemical sensitivity masquerades as common symptoms. It then explores the many causes and cures of chemical sensitivity, chronic Candidiasis, brain fog or toxic encephalopathy, and other "impossible to heal" medical labels.

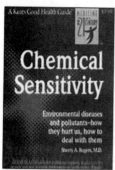

Chemical Sensitivity. This 48-page booklet is the most concise referenced booklet on chemical sensitivity. It is for the person wanting to learn about it, but who is leery of tackling a big book. It is ideal for teaching your physician or convincing your insurance company, as it is fully referenced. And it is a good reference for the veteran who wants a quick concise review.

Most people have difficulty envisioning chemical sensitivity as a potential cause of everyday maladies. But the fact is that a lack of knowledge of the mechanism of chemical sensitivity can be the solo reason that holds many back from ever healing completely. Some will never get truly well, simply because they do not comprehend the tremendous role chemical sensitivity plays. For failure to address the role that chemical sensitivity plays in every disease has been pivotal in failure to get well. The principles of environmental controls are of especially vital importance for cancer victims.

If you are not completely well, you need to read this booklet. If you have been sentenced to a lifetime of drugs, whether it be for high blood pressure, high cholesterol, angina, arrhythmia, asthma, eczema, sinusitis, colitis, learning disabilities, chronic pain or cancer, you need this booklet. It matters not what your label is. What matters is whether chemical sensitivity is a factor that no one has explored that is keeping you from getting well. Most probably it is, and this is an inexpensive way to start you on the path toward drug-free wellness. Then give one to your physician and friends who need to learn about pervasive everyday chemicals and their power to cause disease.

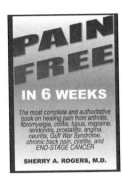

The most complete and authoritative book on healing pain from arthritis, fibromyalgia, colitis, lupus, migraine, tendonitis, prostatitis, angina, neuritis, Gulf War Syndrome, chronic back pain, cystitis, and END-STAGE CANCER

SHERRY A. ROGERS, M.D.

Pain Free in 6 Weeks. All pain has a cause, and once you know the cause, you have the cure. We don't all just look different; we have different chemistries and different underlying causes for our pain.

Old injuries, old age, autoimmune disease, chronic degeneration and even cancer are not the *reasons* for pain. They are mere *labels and excuses* for not finding the true cause and getting rid of it. In fact, the very medications prescribed for pain actually cause deterioration of bone and cartilage, guaranteeing that hip and knee replacement will be needed in the future. They also cause heart disease and many other deadly diseases. But total cure from pain need not be difficult, for the solution may be as simple as eliminating an unidentified food antigen, correcting a nutrient deficiency, healing the gut, or killing an unidentified infection.

For others it has required getting rid of a lifetime's accumulation of everyday toxic chemicals. U.S. EPA studies of chemicals stored in the fat of humans showed that 100% of people harbor environmental chemicals that trigger mysterious back pain, hip pain, arthritis, osteoporosis, painful burning skin, migraines, prostatitis, fibromyalgia, sciatica, degenerating back discs, cystitis, neuropathies, tic doloreau, and even end-stage cancer. When folks get symptoms, they are told that they are a normal consequence of aging, and that there is no known cause or cure. This is totally wrong, as the over 500 scientific references prove. The exciting part is that the majority of folks have total power over their pain. Are you ready to reverse years of pain and become truly **pain free**?

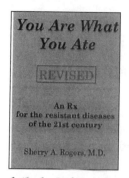

You Are What You Ate

REVISED

An Rx
for the resistant diseases
of the 21st century

Sherry A. Rogers, M.D.

You Are What You Ate. This book is indispensable as the primer and introduction to the macrobiotic diet. The macrobiotic diet is the specialized diet with which many have healed the impossible, including end-stage metastatic cancers. This is after medicine had given up on them and they had been given only months or weeks to live. Yes, they have rallied after surgery, chemotherapy and radiation had failed. Life was seemingly, hopelessly over.

Understandably, this diet has also enabled many chemically sensitive universal reactors, and highly allergic and even "undiagnosable people" to heal. It has also enabled those to heal who have "wastebasket" diagnostic labels such as chronic fatigue, fibromyalgia, MS (multiple sclerosis), rheumatoid arthritis, depression, chronic infections, colitis, asthma, migraines, lupus, chronic Candidiasis, and much more.

Although there are many books on macrobiotics, this is one that takes the special needs of the allergic person and those with multiple food and chemical sensitivities as well as chronic Candidiasis into account. It provides details and case histories that the person new to macrobiotics needs before he embarks on the strict healing phase, as meticulously described in ***The Cure is in the Kitchen***.

Even people who have done the macrobiotic diet for a while will find reasons why they have failed and tips to improve their success. When a diet such as this has allowed many to heal their cancers, any other condition "should be a piece of cake".

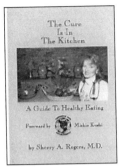

The Cure is in the Kitchen is the next book you should read after *You Are What You Ate* to fully understand how to successfully implement the healing macrobiotic diet. It is the first book to ever spell out in detail what all those people ate day to day who cleared their incurable diseases like MS, rheumatoid arthritis, fibromyalgia, lupus, chronic fatigue, colitis, asthma, migraines, depression, hypertension, heart disease, angina, undiagnosable symptoms, and relentless chemical, food, Candida, and electromagnetic sensitivities, as well as terminal cancers.

Dr. Rogers flew to Boston each month to work side by side with Mr. Michio Kushi, as he counseled people at the end of their medical ropes. As their remarkable case histories will show you, nothing is hopeless. Many of these people had failed to improve with surgery, chemotherapy and radiation. Instead their metastases continued to spread. It was only when they were sent home to die within a few weeks that they turned to the diet.

Medical studies confirm that this diet has more than tripled the survival from cancers. And the beauty of this diet is that you use God-given whole foods to coax the body into the healing mode. It does not rely on prescription drugs, but allows the individual to heal himself at home.

If you cannot afford a $500 consultation, and you choose not to accept your death sentence or medication sentence, why not learn first hand what these people did and how you, too, may improve your health and heal the impossible.

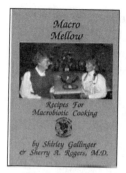

Macro Mellow is a book designed for 4 types of people: (1) For the person who doesn't know a thing about macrobiotics, but just plain wants to cook and eat better to feel better, in spite of the 21st century. (2) It solves the high cholesterol/triglycerides problem without drugs, and is the preferred diet for heart disease patients. In fact, it is the only proven diet to dissolve cholesterol deposits from arterial walls. (3) It is the perfect transition diet for those not ready for macro, but needing to get out of the chronic illness rut. (4) It spells out how to feed the rest of the family members who hate macro, while another family member must eat it in order to clear "incurable" symptoms.

It shows how to convert the "grains, greens, and beans", strict macro food, into delicious "American-looking" food that the kids will eat. This saves the cook from making double meals while one person heals. The delicious low-fat whole food meals designed by Shirley Gallinger, a veteran nurse who has worked with Dr. Rogers for over two decades, uses macro ingredients without the rest of the family even knowing. It is the first book to dovetail creative meal planning, menus, recipes and even gardening so the cook isn't driven crazy.

Most likely your kitchen contains a plethora of cookbooks. But you owe it to yourself and your family to learn how to incorporate healing whole foods, low in fat and high in phyto-nutrients into their diets. Who you have planning and cooking your meals has been proven to be as important if not more important, than who you have chosen for your doctor. Medical research has proven time after time the power of whole food diets to heal where high tech medicines and surgery have failed.

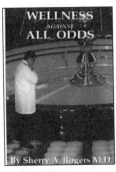

Wellness Against All Odds is a most revolutionary book by Sherry A. Rogers, M.D. It contains the ultimate healing plan that people have successfully used to beat cancer when they were given 2 weeks, some even 2 days to live by esteemed medical centers. These people had exhausted all that medicine has to offer, including surgery, chemotherapy, radiation and bone marrow transplants. Some had even been macrobiotic failures. And one of the most unbelievable things is that the plan costs practically nothing to implement and most of it can be done at home with non-prescription items.

Of course, in keeping with the other works and going far beyond, this contains the mechanisms of how these principles heal and is complete with the scientific references for physicians.   In fact, this program has been proven to more than quadruple cancer survival in the most hopeless forms of cancer (Gonzales, *Nutrition & Cancer*, 33(2): 117-124, 1999).

Did you know, for example, that Harvard physicians have shown how vitamins actually cure some cancers, and over 50 papers in the best medical journals prove it? Likewise, did you know that there are non-prescription enzymes that dissolve cancer, arteriosclerotic plaque, and auto-antibodies like lupus and rheumatoid? Did you know that there is a simple inexpensive, but highly effective way to detoxify the body at home to stop the toxic side effects of chemotherapy within minutes? Did you know that this procedure can also reduce chemical sensitivity reactions (from accidental chemical exposures) from 4 days to 20 minutes? Did you know that there are many hidden causes for "undiagnosable" symptoms that are never looked for, because it is easier and quicker to prescribe a pill than find (and fix) the causes?

The fact is that when you get the body healthy enough, it can heal anything. You do not have to die from labelitis. It no longer matters what your label is, from chronic Candida, fatigue, MS, or chronic pain to chemical sensitivity, an undiagnosable condition, or the worst cancer with only days to survive. If you have been told there is nothing more that can be done for you, you have the option of kicking death in the teeth and healing the impossible. Are you game? And if you can give only one book to a friend with cancer, this is it.

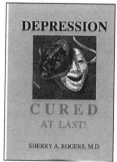

Depression Cured at Last! Just when you think all has been accomplished, along comes one of the most important books of all. Unique in many ways, (1) it is written for the lay person and the physician, and is appropriate as a medical school textbook. In fact, it should be required reading for all physicians regardless of specialty.

(2) It shows that it borders on malpractice to treat depression as a Prozac deficiency, to drug cardiology patients, or any other medical/psychiatric problems without first ruling out proven causes.

With over 700 pages and 1,000 complete references, it covers the **environmental, nutritional** and **metabolic** causes of all disease. It covers leaky gut syndrome, intestinal dysbiosis, hormone deficiencies, hidden sensitivities to foods, molds, and chemicals, dysfunctional detoxication, heavy metal and pesticide poisonings, xenobiotic accumulations, and much, much more.

It is the best blueprint for figuring out what is wrong and how to fix it once and for all. If no one knows what is wrong with you, you need this book. If they know, but say there is no cure, you need this book. If they say you need medications to control your symptoms indefinitely, you need this book. For it is the protocol for the environmental medicine work-up for all disease: how to systematically find the causes.

It is inconceivable that there is anyone who would not benefit from this book, as it surely leaves drug-oriented medicine in the dust of the 20th century. And it does so by using the only disease that by definition sports a lack of hope. We chose this disease, depression, as a prototype, to be sure to drive home the message that just when you least expect it, there is always **hope**. Every symptom has a cause and a cure. Come learn how to find the causes of yours.

Scientific Basis for Selected Environmental Medicine Techniques contains the scientific evidence and references for the techniques of environmental medicine. It is designed with the patient in mind who is being denied medical payments by insurance companies that refuse to acknowledge environmental medicine.

With this guide a patient may choose to represent himself in small claims court and quote from the book showing, for example, that the *Journal of the American Medical Association* states that "titration provides a useful and effective measure of patient sensitivity". Or he may need to prove to his HMO that a U.S. Government agency states that "an exposure history should be taken for every patient". Failure to do so can lead to an inappropriate diagnosis and treatment.

It has sections showing medical references of how finding hidden vitamin deficiencies have, for example, enabled people to heal carpal tunnel syndrome without surgery, or heal life threatening steroid-resistant vasculitis, or stop seizures, or migraines, or learning disabilities.

This book is designed for patients who choose to find the causes of their illnesses, rather than merely mask their symptoms with drugs for the rest of their lives. It is also for those who have been unfairly denied insurance coverage, or appropriate diagnosis by an HMO that is more concerned about profit than finding the cause of their patients' symptoms. And it is the ideal book with which to educate your PTA, attorney, insurance company, or physicians who still doubt your sanity.

In this era, HMO's tell people what diseases they can have, how long they can have them, and what treatments they can have. And all diseases seem to be deficiencies of drugs, for that is how they are all treated. It is as though arthritis were an Advil deficiency. This book arms you with the ammunition to defend your right to find the causes and get rid of symptoms and drugs.

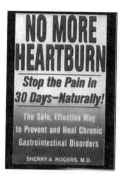

No More Heartburn. The chance of healing any condition in the body is slim to none until the gut is healthy first. Heartburn, indigestion, irritable bowel, spastic colon, colitis, gall bladder disease, gas and bloating are far from benign, for they are all signs of an ailing gastro-intestinal tract. And disease and death began in the gut.

Learn how the many prescription and over-the-counter drugs guarantee that you will not only have worse gut symptoms eventually, but that you can pile on new symptoms, seemingly unrelated to the gut, within the next few years like arthritis, heart problems or cancer.

Come learn how to find the many hidden causes of symptoms like food allergies, Candida overgrowth, Helicobacter, leaky gut, nutrient deficiencies, toxic environment and thoughts, and more. Then learn how to use non-prescription remedies to heal, not merely mask every symptom from mouth to rectum.

Since the gut houses over half the immune system and over half the detoxification system, a silently ailing gut holds back healing any condition indefinitely. This book is also full of new non-prescription Candida and other yeast fighters and protocols, since this is a common unsuspected cause of many diseases.

Learn how heartburn masked with drugs is a fast road to a heart attack or cancer, chronic fatigue, chronic pain or fibromyalgia. Explicit clear directions are given for every gut symptom, their causes and cures. For an unhealthy gut is a primary reason for many folks to be stuck at a standstill, unable to heal any further. If your healing is stalled, chances are you need to start healing the gut first. You need to heal from the inside out, for **the road to health is paved with good intestines.** (Over 350 references)

265

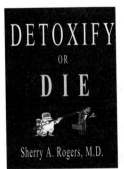

DETOXIFY
OR
DIE

Sherry A. Rogers, M.D.

Detoxify or Die. If you don't own this best-selling book, you're missing out on the most surefire and thoroughly documented way to heal the impossible and reverse aging, regardless of how "stuck" you might feel. Environmental toxins are ubiquitous, impossible to escape. For example, the phthalates from plastic wrap of foods to Styrofoam trays and cups, plastic bottles for water, soda, juices and infant formula leach into our foods. Once inside our bodies they can create any disease and indefinitely stall the chemistry of healing. EPA studies show this pollutant is in every person and is thousands of times more plentiful than the hundreds of other environmental toxins that insidiously stockpile in the body, taking sometimes decades to produce disease seemingly overnight. Luckily there are a multitude of ways to boost your body's ability to detoxify them, starting with the *detox cocktail* that you can make at home every day.

Our lifetime accumulation of pesticides, volatile organic hydrocarbons, heavy metals and more contribute to every disease and symptom. The most exciting part is the proof that getting rid of environmental toxins reverses diseases for which medicine claims there is no known cause and no known cure! Contrast this with medicine's solution that consists of a lifetime sentencing to costly medications with a laundry list of side effects. Once you peel away the underlying causes the body is able to heal itself and disease melts away, as scientific studies in leading medical journals from the Mayo Clinic, for example, clearly prove. Detoxification is equally crucial for the addicted individual trying to get free from alcohol or addiction to prescription or street drugs. This is the most thorough program for medical detoxification, showing you how to do it safely at home, avoiding the pitfalls. The Resources chapter is complete with where to find everything in this book, 1-800 numbers, addresses, web sites and more, plus over 700 complete scientific references. If you buy only one book this year, make it ***Detoxify or Die.***

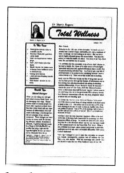

Total Wellness Newsletter

For over a decade and a half, this referenced monthly newsletter has kept folks and physicians up to date on new findings. Since Dr. Rogers is constantly researching, lecturing around the globe, maintaining a private practice, doing television and radio shows, writing for health magazines and physicians, and has published over 20 scientific papers and over 14 books in 15 years, she is peddling as fast as she can.

There is literally an avalanche of new information, but we don't want you to have to wait for a new book on the subject to learn about it. We want that practical and useful new instruction in your hands every month.

Furthermore, the field of environmental medicine, because it is so all encompassing, can be overwhelming at times. So in addition to bringing you the new, we also focus on the overall perspective as well as the practical solutions you can do today.

In this era, because we cannot get the information out to you fast enough, we use the newsletter as our communication link. By sending you to the medical school of the future each month, *Total Wellness* will teach you useful facts years before they will be presented elsewhere, and it is practical and action-oriented, giving you explicit directions and sources. For pennies a day you really cannot afford to be without this life-altering, money saving unique information.

We continually receive kind letters that read, "I had to laugh last week when all the newspapers and television shows were abuzz with the hot new medical discovery. If they had been readers of your newsletter, they could have learned about it 10 years ago, as I did!"

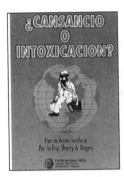

Cansancio o Intoxicacion?

(*Tired or Toxic?* in Spanish) El lego informado reconoce que a medida que el mundo se vuelve más tecnológico, el hombre pierde proporcionalmente más control sobre su vida. Este libro le permitirá recuperar el control de su salud, ofreciéndole mayor capacidad para formar equipo con su medico para diagnosticar y tratar su condición.

Esta información es vitalmente importante ahora ya que a todos toca con cualquier síntoma tal como la sensibilidad química, alto colesterol, fatiga crónica, complejo relacionado a Cándida, depresion, Alzheimer, hipertensión, diabetes, enfermedad cardíaca, osteoporosis y más.

Dra. Rogers se encuentra en la avanazada de la educación pública sobre los efectos del medio ambiente en el individuo.

Otros libros escritos por Dra. Rogers que tienen que ver con prevenir enfermedades y restablecer la salud son **Eres lo que Has Comido, El Síndrome de E.A.,** y **La Cura Se Encuentra En La Cocina:** La Fase Curativa Estricta de la Dieta Macrobiotica.

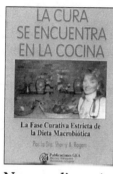

La Fase Curativa Estricta de
la Dieta Macrobiótica

Por la Dra. Sherry A. Rogers

Publicaciones GEA

La Cura Se Encuentra En La Cocina
(*The Cure Is In The Kitchen* in Spanish)
Este libro explora la relación entre dieta, medio ambiente, salud, y enfermedad y explica como la dieta macrobiótica, basada en cereales integrales, porotos y sus productos y otros alimentos naturales integrales puede prevenir enfermedades y restablecer la salud.

Nos explica cómo una dieta muy artificial contribuye a una variedad de problemas de salud y cómo ciertos aspectos de la vida moderna también nos pueden debilitar.

Un programa macrobiótico consiste de dos fases; pasar gradualmente a una dieta macrobótica o ponerse en una fase curativa estricta de carácter temporario. El objectivo de la fase curativa de esta dieta es aclarar una condición en particular. Es necesariamente, muy estricta e individualizada, y por eso razón, la persona debe consultar un doctor entrenado en la macrobiótica.

Otros libros escritos por Dra. Rogers que tienen que ver con prevenir enfermedades y restablecer la salud son **Cansancio o Intoxicación?, Eres lo que Has Comido,** y **El Síndrome de E.A.**

Mold Plates: An Investment in Your Future Health

Mold is unavoidably ubiquitous and an unsuspected cause of many illnesses, whether common, "incurable" or mysterious. In fact one reason why many insurance companies deny coverage for mold-related damage now may be in part because it can mimic any symptoms you can name. We used to think of mold as just a cause of only typical allergic symptoms like post nasal drip, sinusitis, migraines, headaches, dizziness, ringing in the ears, recurrent soar throats, exhaustion, burning eyes, itchy eyes, bronchitis, asthma, chronic cough, eczema, hives, and more. But now colitis, arthritis, depression, schizophrenia, learning disorders, rare neurologic problems, and even behavior mimicking brain injury can be added to the list of mold mimics.

Since mold is a common, yet remedial cause of symptoms, you first need to know if you have too much. By exposing special petri dishes (or mold plates) in your bedroom, family room, and office, you have effectively assessed your 24 hour mold environment.

Each plate comes with directions for exposure and as well as instructions to enable you to assess the amount of mold contamination you have by interpreting your own mold plates. You'll need to order one plate for each room you want to assess at home or work.

You may have an air filter that is not removing sufficient mold, or a home structural problem with hidden leaks contributing to sustained mold levels. A mold plate with a special agar that yields 30% more growth can demonstrate this. Since mold is not static, but constantly growing, you may need to periodically assess the contribution it is making to your environment, symptoms and life.

If you do not know how many molds is in your environment, you may erroneously be attributing symptoms to chemical or food sensitivities or just settling for "It's undiagnosable and untreatable". It is always best to meet the unseen enemy head on to optimally identify the cause of the problem and to be able to solve it, once and for all.

Personal Phone Consultations with Dr. Rogers

Many people are stuck. They have an undiagnosable condition. Or they have a label but have been unable to get well. Or they have a "dead-end" label that means nothing more can be done. And many are not able to find a physician who is trained in what our books explore, and need for example, help in interpreting their laboratory results.

These people could benefit from a personal consultation with Sherry Rogers, M.D. to explore what diagnostic and treatment options may exist that they or their physicians are not aware of. For this reason we offer prepaid, scheduled phone consultations with the doctor. These can be scheduled through the office by calling (315) 488-2856.

If you wish to send copies of your medical reports and/or also have your doctor or spouse on the line, this can be helpful as well. Reports must be received at least 3 weeks prior to the consult and not be on fax paper. They should be copies and not originals as they are not returnable. Do not send records without first having secured a scheduled appointment time, for records without an appointment are discarded.

Because you have not come to the office and been examined, you are not considered a patient. In spite of that, you can learn what tests your physician could order and what plans you could follow. If you need help in interpreting tests, a scheduled follow-up consultation can allow you to explore treatment options with specific nutrient and other treatment suggestions. The point is, you do not have to be alone without guidance in your quest for wellness. And you owe it to yourself to explore the options that you might otherwise never even have heard of.

PRESTIGE PUBLISHING
1-800-846-6687 ◊ Fax 315-454-8119
www.prestigepublishing.com

Price List

The High Blood Pressure Hoax	$19.95
Detoxify or Die	$22.95
Depression Cured At Last!	$24.95
The E.I. Syndrome Revised	$17.95
Tired or Toxic?	$18.95
Chemical Sensitivity (booklet)	$ 3.95
You Are What You Ate	$12.95
The Cure Is In The Kitchen	$14.95
Macro Mellow	$12.95
Wellness Against All Odds	$17.95
The Scientific Basis for Environmental Medicine Techniques	$17.95
No More Heartburn	$15.00
Pain-Free In 6 Weeks	$19.95

Spanish Translations

Cansancio o Intoxicacion?	$30.00
La Cura Se Encuentra En La Cocina	$30.00

Newsletter

Total Wellness Newsletter

Monthly referenced newsletter on current wellness and healing information/1 year (12 issues, 8 pages per issue)	$39.95
Back issues/1 year (12 issues, 8 pages per issue)	$29.95
Back issues/each	$ 4.00

Services

Mold Plates (one room)	$25.00

Phone Consultations

Telephone consultations available with Dr. Rogers. Contact Dr. Rogers office (315) 488-2856 for scheduling information.

Index

8

8-OhdG, 44, 56, 220

A

Accelerated aging, 9, 30, 83, 87, 170, 202, 208
Accelerated heavy metal detox, 94, 108, 111
Accupril, 15, 171
ACE inhibitors, 15, 171
ACES with Zinc, 21, 22, 195, 219
Acetyl L-Carnitine, 44, 48, 56, 71, 219
Acetyl-L-Carnitine or ALC, 43, 61
Acidity, 163, 165, 166
Acidosis, 163, 164
Acrylic, 127
Adhesives, 126, 127
ADMA, 31, 32, 33, 56, 183, 189, 220
Adrenal, 128, 189, 190, 191, 192
Adrenal Stress Profile, 191, 220, 225
Aging, 9, 10, 17, 19, 21, 30, 38, 41, 42, 43, 44, 45, 46, 47, 48, 52, 54, 61, 71, 78, 79, 83, 87, 104, 122, 140, 141, 151, 164, 166, 170, 184, 186, 190, 192, 202, 208, 229, 230, 258, 266
Air purifier, 122
Alcohol, 141, 145, 266
Aldomet, 16
Aldoril, 16
Alkaline water, 34, 162, 164, 168
Alkaline Water Machine, a.k.a. Spring Ionizer, 164, 166, 168, 175, 220
Allergies, 3, 123, 173, 265
Alpha-tocopherol, 39, 53, 59, 61
Altace, 15, 171
American Environmental Health Foundation, 224, 251
Aneurysm, 3
Anger, 145, 234, 246, 251
Angina, 3, 6, 29, 62, 68, 94, 116, 119, 145, 187, 188, 215, 257, 260

Antioxidant, 34, 36, 38, 45, 48, 50, 52, 54, 57, 58, 59, 61, 85, 151, 152, 153, 154, 166, 167, 169, 176, 177, 178, 193, 230, 232
Apresaline, 16
Argentyn 23, 85, 86, 87
Arginine, 30, 32, 33, 34, 56, 57, 63, 209, 214
Arrhythmia, 3, 6, 9, 32, 36, 136, 212, 257
Arsenic, 93, 95, 103, 110
Arthritis, 3, 7, 16, 73, 78, 79, 158, 173, 183, 196, 201, 204, 206, 258, 259, 260, 264, 265, 270
Aspirin, 36, 62
Asthma, 6, 257, 259, 260, 270
Asymmetrical dimethyl arginine, 31, 57
Atheromatous plaque, 77
Atrial fibrillation, 36, 188

B

Band-Aid, 51, 52, 83, 166
B-Complete-100, 106, 131
Benign prostatic hypertrophy BPH, 79
Beta-Blockers, 14, 193
Bile Acid Factors, 71, 87
BioSil, 78, 109, 131
Birdseed cereal, 146, 154, 157, 158, 159
Blood clots, 39, 76, 81, 215
Blood pressure cuff Sphygmomanometer, 3
Blood vessels, broken, 2
Boron, 79, 108, 109, 131, 209, 220
Boxed breakfast cereals, 155
Brain shrinking, 11, 143
Brassica, 129, 160, 161
Breast cancer, 90, 156, 188, 198, 201, 210, 229, 251
Broccoli seeds, 161
Buckwheat, 146, 153, 154, 157, 158
Buffering, 163, 164, 165

273

C

D

W

Z